Baillière's
Abbreviations
in Medicine

KU-642-870

Baillière's Abbreviations in Medicine

Edwin B. Steen, PhD

Professor Emeritus of Anatomy and Physiology
Western Michigan University

Fifth Edition

Baillière Tindall
London Philadelphia Toronto

Baillière Tindall   1 St Anne's Road
Eastbourne, East Sussex BN21 3UN
England

West Washington Square
Philadelphia, PA 19105, USA

1 Goldthorne Avenue
Toronto, Ontario M8Z 5T9, Canada

First published 1960
Fourth edition 1978
Fifth edition 1984
  Reprinted 1985

Typeset by Central Southern Typesetters, Eastbourne
Printed and bound in Great Britain by William Clowes Ltd,
Beccles and London

British Library Cataloguing in Publication Data

Steen, Edwin B.
  Baillière's abbreviations in medicine—5th ed.
  1. Medicine—Abbreviations
  I. Title   II. Steen, Edwin B. Abbreviations in
  medicine
  610′.148   R123

  ISBN 0–7020–1036–7

Contents

Preface

It was apparent several years ago that the widespread use of abbreviations in medical literature had reached a point where a handy source of reference had become a necessity. The original edition of this dictionary, the first of its kind in the field of medicine and the related sciences, was published in the United States in 1960 in the hope that it would fulfil that need and, at the same time, help to introduce a measure of standardization into an otherwise chaotic field. The success of that edition, and of its successors, has now led to the need for a fifth edition.

The scope of the dictionary has been extensively widened by adding new abbreviations from nearly every field of medicine. These include additional abbreviations of medical organizations, terms used in dentistry, occupational and physical therapy, cardiorespiratory therapy, and other specialized fields. Abbreviations of many new biochemical terms now used in medicine have been added. Especial attention has been given to the inclusion of new abbreviations employed in various laboratory procedures and reports and in the everyday operation of hospitals and clinics.

Because of the large number of new abbreviations encountered in the preparation of this revision, a degree of selection had to be employed as not all could be included. Abbreviations for short words, except for weights and measures, have been omitted as well as abbreviations for trite or trivial terms. Multiple abbreviations for the same term have been reduced in number. (Although this book is not a list of 'correct' usage, the preferred SI abbreviation is indicated.) Some abbreviations for highly specialized terms having a restricted use are not listed. Abbreviations for terms identifying structures in illustrations appearing in texts or scientific papers are generally omitted.

Full stops separating the letters have been omitted from entries in line with the current trend of writing abbreviations without stops, and to avoid duplication (and pontification) where both styles are employed.

Abbreviations are given throughout the book in capitals except where common usage dictates the use of small letters. Needless to say, where there is any possibility of confusion in the context, words should be spelled out in full. The use of italic has been reserved for Latin terms defined in the dictionary and for scientific names of organisms.

I should like to thank those who have aided in the revision by calling attention to errors and suggesting new abbreviations to be listed. Especially appreciated were the contributions of Dr Adam G. N. Moore of Boston, Mass. and Dr R. J. Hetherington of Birmingham, England. I am grateful also to the Upjohn Company, Bronson Methodist Hospital, the Borgess Hospital, and Western Michigan University, all of Kalamazoo, Michigan, and to the editorial staff of my publishers for their contributions and helpful suggestions.

Edwin B. Steen   *February 1984*

A

A absorbance (symbol for in spectrophotometry); acceptor; accommodation; acetum; adenine; adenosine; adrenaline; adult; akinetic; allergy, allergist; alveolar gas; ampere (SI); amphetamine; ampicillin; anaesthetic; anaphylaxis; Ångström unit; *annum* (L) year; anterior; aqueous; area (of heart shadow); argon; arteria; atrium; auricle; *auris* (L) ear

a accommodation; acid; acidity, total; ampere; anode; anterior; *aqua* (L) water; area; artery; asymmetric; atto (prefix); axial

α alpha; Symbol designating *first;* In organic compounds, refers to the carbon atom which is next to the carbon atom bearing the active group of molecules

Å Ångström unit

A II angiotensin II

A₂ aortic second sound

AA achievement age; Alcoholics Anonymous; amino acid; amyloid-A protein; anticipatory avoidance; arachidonic acid; Association of Anaesthetists

āā, āa *ana* (Gr) of each

AAA abdominal aortic aneurysm; acute anxiety attack; American Academy of Allergy; American Academy of Anatomists

aaa amalgam

AAAHE American Association for the Advancement of Health Education

AAALAC American Association for Accreditation of Laboratory Animal Care

AAAS American Association for the Advancement of Science

AABB American Association of Blood Banks

AAC antimicrobial agents and chemotherapy

AACCN American Association of Critical Care Nurses

AACHP American Association for Comprehensive Health Planning

AACP American Association of Colleges of Pharmacy

AACPDM American Academy for Cerebral Palsy and Developmental Medicine

AAD alloxazine adenine dinucleotide (FAD)

AADP American Academy of Dental Prosthetics; amyloid A-degrading protease

AADR American Academy of Dental Radiology

AADS American Association of Dental Schools

AAE active assistive exercise; acute allergic encephalitis; American Association of Endodontists

AAEH Association to Advance Ethical Hypnosis

AAF acetic-alcohol-formalin; acetylaminofluorine; Army Air Force; ascorbic acid factor

AAFP American Academy of Family Physicians

AAGP American Academy of General Practice; American Association for Geriatric Psychiatry

AAHD American Association of Hospital Dentists

AAHE Association for the Advancement of Health Education

AAHPER American Academy for Health, Physical Education and Recreation

AAI American Association of Immunologists

AAID American Academy of Implant Dentistry

AAIN American Association of Industrial Nurses

AAL anterior axillary line

AALAS American Association of Laboratory Animal Science

AAMA American Academy of Medical Administrators

AAMC American Association of Medical Clinics; American Association of Medical Colleges

AAMFT American Association for Marriage and Family Therapy

AAMI Association for the Advancement of Medical Instrumentation

AAMIH American Association for Maternal and Infant Health

AAMMC American Association of Medical Milk Commissioners

AAMP American Academy of Medical Preventics

AAMR American Academy of Mental Retardation

AAMRL American Association of Medical Record Librarians

AAN American Academy of Neurology; American Academy of Nursing; American Academy of Nutrition

AANA American Association of Nurse Anesthetists

AANM American Association of Nurse-Midwives

AANPI American Association of Nurses Practicing Independently

AAO American Academy of Ophthalmology; American Academy of Optometry; American Academy of Osteopathy; American Association of Ophthalmologists; American Association of Orthodontists; amino acid oxidase

AAofA Ambulance Association of America

AAOO American Academy of Ophthalmology and Otolaryngology

AAOP American Academy of Oral Pathology

AAOS American Academy of Orthopedic Surgeons

AAP American Academy of Pediatrics; American Academy of Periodontology; American Academy of Psychoanalysts; American Academy of Psychotherapists; American Association of Pathologists; Association for the Advancement of Psychoanalysis; Association for the Advancement of Psychotherapy; Association of American Physicians

AAPA American Association of Physicians' Assistants

AAPB American Association of Pathologists and Bacteriologists

AAPHD American Association of Public Health Dentists

AAPHP American Association of Public Health Physicians

AAPMC antibiotic-associated pseudomembranous colitis

AAPMR American Association of Physical Medicine and Rehabilitation

AAPS Association of American Physicians and Surgeons; American Association of Plastic Surgeons

AART American Association for Rehabilitation Therapy; American Association for Respiratory Therapy

AAS American Academy of Sanitarians; anthrax antiserum; aortic arch syndrome

AASD American Academy of Stress Disorders

AASH adrenal androgen stimulating hormone

AASP American Association of Senior Physicians

AAT alanine aminotransferase; alpha-antitrypsin; auditory apperception test

AATS American Association for Thoracic Surgery

AAVMC Association of American Veterinary Medical Colleges

AAVP American Association of Veterinary Parasitologists

AB abortion; Aid to the Blind; antigen-binding; apex beat; *Artium Baccalaureus* (L) Bachelor of Arts; asthmatic bronchitis; axiobuccal

A>B air greater than bone (conduction)

Ab antibody

ab abortion; about; antibody

ABA abscissic acid; allergic bronchopulmonary aspergillosis

abbr abbreviation(-iated)

ABC aconite, belladonna, chloroform; antigen-binding capacity; airway, breathing, and circulation (cardiopulmonary resuscitation); atomic, biological, chemical (warfare); axiobuccocervical

ABCC Atomic Bomb Casualty Commission

ABCIL antibody-mediated cell-dependent immune lympholysis

ABD aged, blind, disabled

abd abdomen (-dominal); abduction (-ductor)

abdom abdomen (-dominal)

ABE acute bacterial endocarditis

abe abequose residue

ABG arterial blood gases; axiobuccogingival

ABL axiobuccolingual; Army Biological Laboratory; Automated Biological Laboratory

Abn abnormal

abnor abnormal

ABO absent bed occupancy

Abor abortion

ABP androgen-binding protein; arterial blood pressure

ABPA allergic bronchopulmonary aspergillosis

ABR Abortus Bang Ringprobe (test); absolute bed rest

ABr agglutination test for brucellosis

abras abrasions

ABS acute brain syndrome; alkylbenzyl sulphonates

abs absent; absolute

abs feb *absente febre* (L) in the absence of fever

abstr abstract

abt about

ABVD adriamycin, bleomycin, vinblastine, and dacarbazine

ABY acid bismuth yeast (agar)

AC abdominal circumference; acetylcholine; Acupuncture Clinic (Brit); acute; adrenal cortex or corticoid; air conduction; all culture (broth); alternating current; anodal closure; anticomplementary; anti-inflammatory corticoid; atriocarotid; auriculocarotid; axiocervical

Ac accelerator (e.g. *Ac-globulin*); acetyl; acryl group

ac acute; *ante cibum* (L) before meals

ACA American Chiropractic Association; American College of Allergists; American College of Anesthesiologists; American College of Angiology; American College of Apothecaries; American Council on Alcoholism; automatic clinical analyser

ACACN American Council of Applied Clinical Nutrition

acad academy

ACB antibody-coated bacteria

ACBG aorta-coronary bypass graft

ACC anodal closure contraction; acinic cell carcinoma; adrenocortical carcinoma

Acc adenoid cystic carcinoma

acc acceleration; accident; accommodation; according

AcCh acetylcholine

AcChR acetylcholine receptor

accid accident(al)

ACCL anodal closure clonus

AcCoA acetyl coenzyme A

accom accommodation

ACCP American College of Chest Physicians; American College of Clinical Pharmacology

accur *accuratissime* (L) most carefully, accurately

ACD absolute cardiac dullness; acid citrate dextrose (solution); American College of Dentists; anterior chest diameter

AC-DC bisexual (homosexual and heterosexual)

ACD sol citric acid, trisodium citrate, dextrose solution

ACE acetonitrile; adrenal cortical extract; alcohol-chloroform-ether (mixture)

ACEH acid cholesterol ester hydrolase

ACEP American College of Emergency Physicians

ACF accessory clinical findings; Acute Care Facility

ACFO American College of Foot Orthopedists

ACFS American College of Foot Surgeons

ACG American College of Gastroenterology; angiocardiography; apex cardiogram

AcG accelerator globulin (factor V)

ACGME Accreditation Council on Graduate Medical Education

ACGP American College of General Practitioners

ACGPOMS American College of General Practitioners in Osteopathic Medicine and Surgery

ACH adrenal cortical hormone; arm, chest, height; arm girth, chest depth, hip width (index of nutrition)

ACh acetylcholine

ACHA American College of Hospital Administrators

AChE acetylcholinesterase

AChR acetylcholine receptor

AChS Association of the Society of Chiropodists

AC&HS before meals and at bedtime

ACI acoustic comfort index; adenylate cyclase inhibitor; anticlonus index

ACIR Automotive Crash Injury Research

ACL anterior cruciate ligament

ACLM American College of Legal Medicine

ACLS Advanced Cardiac Life Support Program

ACME Advisory Council on Medical Education

ACMS American Chinese Medical Society

ACN American College of Neuropsychiatrists; acute conditioned neuroses; American College of Nutrition

ACNM American College of Nuclear Medicine; American College of Nurse-Midwives

ACO American College of Otolaryngologists; anodal closing odour

ACOG American College of Obstetricians and Gynecologists

ACOHA American College of Osteopathic Hospital

Administrators

ACO-HNS American Council of Otolaryngology – Head and Neck Surgery

ACOI American College of Osteopathic Internists

ACOMS American College of Oral and Maxillofacial Surgeons

ACOOG American College of Osteopathic Obstetricians and Gynecologists

ACOP American College of Osteopathic Pediatricians

ACOS American College of Osteopathic Surgeons

acous acoustics, acoustical

ACP acid phosphatase; acyl carrier protein; American College of Pathologists; American College of Pharmacists; American College of Physicians; American College of Prosthodontists; American College of Psychiatrists; Animal Care Panel; anodal closing picture; Association for Child Psychiatrists; Association of Clinical Pathologists; Association of Correctional Psychologists

ACPM American College of Preventative Medicine

ACPP adrenocorticopolypeptide

ACR acriflavine; American College of Radiology; anticonstipation regimen

Acr acrylic

ACS American Cancer Society; American Chemical Society; American College of Surgeons; anodal closing sound; antireticular cytotoxic serum; aperture current setting

ACSM American College of Sports Medicine

ACSP Advisory Council on Scientific Policy

ACT achievement through counselling and treatment; actinomycin; advanced coronary treatment; anticoagulant therapy

act active

ACTA Automatic Computerized Transverse Axial (X-ray system)

act-C actinomycin C

act-D actinomycin D

ACTe anodal closure tetanus

ACTH adrenocorticotrophic hormone

ACTN adrenocorticotrophin

ACTP adrenocorticotrophic polypeptide

AD addict; adenoid degeneration (virus); alcohol dehydrogenase; Alzheimer's disease; analgesic dose; anodal duration; antigenic determinant; arthritic dose; *auris dextra* (L) right ear; Associate Degree (Nursing Programs); autonomic dysreflexia; average deviation; axiodistal; diphenylchlorarsine

Ad adrenal

ad *adde* or *addetur* (L) let them be added; axiodistal

ADA American Dental Association; American Dermatological Association; American Diabetes Association; American Dietetic Association

ADAMHA Alcohol, Drug Abuse and Mental Health Administration

ADAP American Dental Assistant's Program; Assistant Director of Army Psychiatry (Brit)

ADB accidental death benefit

ADC Aid to Dependent Children; albumin, dextrose, catalase (media); ambulance design criteria; anodal duration contraction; axiodistocervical

AdC adrenal cortex

ADCC antibody-dependent cell-mediated cytotoxicity

ADD adenosine deaminase; androstanediene-dione; attention-deficit disorder

add *adde* (L) add; *addantur* (L) let them be added; addition; adduction(-ductor)

add c trit *adde cum tritu* (L) add trituration

ad def an *ad defectionem animi* (L) to the point of fainting

ad deliq *ad deliquium* (L) to fainting

addend *addendus* (L) to be added

addict addiction

addn addition

ADDS American Digestive Disease Society

ADE acute disseminated encephalitis; apparent digestible energy

Ade adenine

Ade Cbl adenosylcobalamin

ad effect *ad effectum* (L) until effectual

ad feb *adstante febre* (L) fever being present

ADG   axiodistogingival

ADGMS   Assistant Director General of Medical Services

ad gr acid   *ad gratum aciditatem* (L) to an agreeable acidity

ad gr gust   *ad gratum gustum* (L) to an agreeable taste

ADH   antidiuretic hormone (vasopressin)

ADHA   American Dental Hygienists' Association

adhib   *adhibendus* (L) to be administered

ADI   Academy of Dentistry, International; acceptable daily intake; axiodistoincisal

ad int   *ad interim* (L) meanwhile

adj   adjunct

ADL   activities of daily living

ad lib   *ad libitum* (L) at pleasure

ADM   adriamycin (doxorubicin)

AdM   adrenal medulla

Adm   admission, admitted

Admin   administer, administration

admov   *admove, admoveatur* (L) apply, let it be applied

ADMS   Assistant Director of Medical Services

ad naus   *ad nauseam* (L) to the extent of producing nausea

ad neut   *ad neutralizandum* (L) to neutralization

ADO   axiodisto-occlusal

ADP   Academy of Dental Prosthetics; Animal Disease and Parasite Research Division (USDA); adenosine diphosphate; automatic data processing

ad part dolent   *ad partes dolentes* (L) to the painful parts

ADPL   average daily patient load

ad pond om   *ad pondus omnium* (L) to the weight of the whole

ADR   Accepted Dental Remedies; adriamycin (doxorubicin); adverse drug reaction

Adr   adrenaline

ADS   American Denture Society; antidiuretic substance; Army Dental Services

ad sat   *ad saturandum* (L) to saturation

adst feb   *adstante febre* (L) when fever is present

ADT   a placebo, meaning A (*any*), D (*what you desire*), T (*thing*); accepted dental therapeutics; agar-gel diffusion test; alternate-day treatment

ADTA American Dental Trade Association

ADTe tetanic contraction

ad us *ad usum* (L) according to custom

ad us ext *ad usum externum* (L) for external use

ADV adenovirus

A/DV arterio/deep venous

adv. *adversum* (L) against, adverse to

ad 2 vic *ad duas vices* (L) at two times, for two doses

A5D5W alcohol 5%, dextrose 5%, in water

ADX adrenalectomized

AE above-elbow; acrodermatosis enteropathica; anoxic encephalopathy; antitoxic unit (German abbreviation for); energy of activation

A+E Accident and Emergency (Ward or Dept); analysis and evaluation

AEA alcohol, ether, acetone (solution); Atomic Energy Authority

AEC at earliest convenience; Atomic Energy Commission

AEE Atomic Energy Establishment

AEG air encephalogram

aeg *aegra* (L) the patient

AEI acrylic eye illustrator

AEM analytical electron microscopy

AEMC Albert Einstein Medical Center

AEMIS Aerospace and Environmental Medicine Information System

AEP artificial endocrine pancreas; auditory evoked potential

AEq age equivalent

aeq *aequales* (L) equal

AER acoustic evoked response; aldosterone excretion rate

AERE Atomic Energy Research Establishment

Aero *Aerobacter*

AES American Encephalographic Society; American Endocrine Society; American Epidemiological Society

AESQ Aeromedical Evacuation Squadron (Air Force)

AEST Aeromedical Evacuation Support Team

aet   *aetas* (L) age aetiology

aetat   *aetatis* (L) age

aetiol   aetiology

AF   abnormal frequency; acid-fast; aflatoxin; Air Force; albumin-free (tuberculin); aldehyde fuchsin; amniotic fluid; angiogenesis factor; Armed Forces; Arthritis Foundation; atrial fibrillation; audio frequency; auricular fibrillation

af   audiofrequency

AFAR   American Foundation for Aging Research

AFB   acid-fast bacillus; aflatoxin B; American foulbrood; aorto-femoral bypass

AFC   antibody-forming cell

AFCR   American Federation for Clinical Research

AFDC   Aid to Families with Dependent Children

aff   afferent; *affinis* (L) having an affinity with but not identical with

AFG   aflatoxin G; amniotic fluid glucose

AFH   Air Force Hospital

AFI   amaurotic familial idiocy

AFib   atrial fibrillation

AFIP   Armed Forces Institute of Pathology

AFL   aflatoxicol; anti-fatty liver (with reference to a factor in pancreatic tissue)

AFM   aflatoxin M

AFML   Armed Forces Medical Library

AFMML   Air Force Medical Materials Letter

AFNC   Air Force Nurse Corps

aFP   alpha-fetoprotein

AFPP   acute fibrinopurulent pneumonia

AFQ   aflatoxin Q

AFQT   Armed Forces Qualification Test

AFR   aqueous flare response; ascorbic free radical

AFRD   acute febrile respiratory disease

AFRI   acute febrile respiratory illness

AFS   American Fertility Society

AFSAM   Air Force School of Aviation Medicine

AFSP   acute fibrinoserous pneumonia

AFT   aflatoxin

AFTA   American Family Therapy Association

AFTC apparent free testosterone concentration

AFTN autonomously functioning thyroid nodule

AG analytical grade (organic chemistry); antiglobulin; antigravity; atrial gallop; axiogingival

A/G ratio albumin-globulin ratio

Ag antigen; silver (L) *argentum*

AGA accelerated growth area; American Gastroenterological Association; American Genetic Association; American Geriatrics Association; American Goiter Association; appropriate for gestational age

Ag-Ab antigen-antibody complex

AGBAD Alexander Graham Bell Association for the Deaf

AGCT Army General Classification Test

AGD agar-gel diffusion; agarose diffusion (method)

AGE angle of greatest extension

AGF angle of greatest flexion

ag feb *aggrediente febre* (L) when the fever increases

AGG agammaglobulinaemia

agg agglutination(-ated); aggregate

aggl agglutination(-ated)

agglut agglutination(-ated)

AGGS anti gas gangrene serum

AGI Alan Guttmacher Institute

AgI silver iodide

agit *agita* (L) shake, stir

agit ante sum *agita ante sumendum* (L) shake before taking

agit vas *agitato vase* (L) the vial being shaken

AGL acute granulocytic leukaemia

AGMK African green monkey kidney

AGN acute glomerulonephritis; agnosia

AgNOR silver-staining nucleolar organizer region

AGOS American Gynecological and Obstetrical Society

AGP acid glycoprotein; agar gel precipitation (test)

AGPA American Group Practice Association; American Group Psychotherapy Association

AGR anticipatory goal response

AGS adrenogenital syndrome

AGT antiglobulin test

agt agent

AGTr adrenoglomerulotrophin

AGTT abnormal glucose tolerance test

AGV aniline gentian violet

AH abdominal hysterectomy; accidental hypothermia; after-hyperpolarization; Army Hospital; arterial hypertension; artificial heart; ascites hepatoma; autonomic hyperreflexia

A+H Accident and Health (Insurance)

Ah hypermetropic astigmatism

AHA American Heart Association; American Hospital Association; anterior hypothalamic area (of brain); aspartyl-hydroxamic acid; Associate, Institute of Hospital Administrators

AHD autoimmune haemolytic disease; arteriosclerotic heart disease

AHDP azacycloheptane-diphosphonate

AHE acute haemorrhagic encephalomyelitis

AHES artificial heart energy system

AHF acute heart failure; American Health Foundation; American Hepatic Foundation; American Hospital Formulary; antihaemophilic factor (Factor VIII); Associated Health Foundation

AHG aggregated human globulin; antihaemophilic globulin; antihuman globulin

AHGS acute herpetic gingival stomatitis

AHH Association for Holistic Health

AHI active hostility index; Animal Health Institute

AHIP Assisted Health Insurance Plan

AHMA American Holistic Medicine Association

AHMC Association of Hospital Management Committees

AHN Army Head Nurse; assistant head nurse

AHP acute haemorrhagic pancreatitis; American Health Professionals; Assistant House Physician

AHPA American Health Planning Association

AHR Association for Health Records

AHRA American Hospital Radiology Administrators

AHRF American Hearing Research Foundation

AHS Academy of Health Sciences (Army); American Hearing Society; American Hospital Society; Assistant House Surgeon

AHSC American Hospital Supply Corp.

AHSN Assembly of Hospital Schools of Nursing

AHT antihyaluronidase titre

AHTG antihuman thymocytic globulin

AHTP antihuman thymocytic plasma

AI accidental injury; angiogenesis inhibitor; anxiety index; aortic incompetence; aortic insufficiency; artificial insemination; atherogenic index; axioincisal

AIA amylase inhibitor activity

AIBA amino-isobutyric acid

AIBS American Insitute of Biological Sciences

AICF autoimmune complement fixation

AID acquired immunodeficiency disease; acute infectious disease; Agency for International Development; artificial insemination by donor (heterologous insemination); autoimmune deficiency; autoimmune disease

AIDS acquired immune deficiency syndrome

AIF anti-invasion factor

AIH American Institute of Homeopathy; artificial insemination by husband (homologous insemination)

AIHA American Industrial Hygiene Association; autoimmune haemolytic anaemia

AIHC American Industrial Health Conference

AIIMS All-India Institute of Medical Sciences

AIL angioimmunoblastic lymphadenopathy

AILD angioimmunoblastic lymphadenopathy with dysproteinaemia

AIM Amputees in Motion; Artificial Intelligence in Medicine

AIMS abnormal involuntary movement scale

AIN American Institute of Nutrition

AInsuf aortic insufficiency

AIP acute intermittent porphyria; aldosterone-induced protein; Anatuberculin, Petragnani's integral; automated immunoprecipitin (system)

AIPS American Institute of Pathologic Science

AIR amino-imidazole ribonucleotide

AIS androgen insensitivity syndrome

AIS/MR Alternative Intermediate Services for the Mentally Retarded

AIU absolute iodine uptake

AJ ankle jerk

AK above knee

AK amp above knee amputation

AL acute leukaemia; adaptation level; alignment mark (cardiography); axiolingual

Al aluminium

al *auris laeva* (L) left ear

ALA American Laryngological Association; American Lung Association; aminolaevulinic acid

ALa axiolabial

Ala alanine

ALaG axiolabiogingival
ALaL axiolabiolingual
Al-Anon Alcoholics Anonymous
alb albumin
albus (L) white
ALC Alternative Lifestyle Checklist; avian leukosis complex; axiolinguocervical
alc alcohol
ALCAR phosphoribosyl-5-amino-imidazole-carboxamide
AlcR alcohol rub
AlCr aluminium crown
Ald aldolase
aldo aldosterone
ALEP atypical lymphoepithelioid cell proliferation
ALF American Liver Foundation
ALG antilymphocyte globulin; axiolinguogingival
alk alkaline
ALL acute lymphoblastic leukaemia
ALLO atypical *Legionella*-like organisms
ALMA Adoptee's Liberty Movement Association
ALMI anterior lateral myocardial infarct
ALO axilinguo-occlusal
ALOS average length of stay (in Health Care Institutions)
ALP alkaline phosphatase; anterior lobe of pituitary
ALROS American Laryngological, Rhinological and Otological Society
ALS Advanced Life Support System; amyotrophic lateral sclerosis; anticipated life span; antilymphocytic serum
ALT alanine aminotransferase; alternate; altitude
ALTB acute laryningotracheobronchitis
alt dieb *alternis diebus* (L) every other day
alt hor *alternis horis* (L) every other hour
alt noc *alternis nocta* (L) every other night
ALV avian leukosis virus
alv alveolar
alv adst *alvo adstricta* (L) when the bowels are constipated
alv deject *alvi dejectiones* (L) discharge from the bowels
Alvx alveolectomy
ALW arch-loop-whorl
AM actomyosin; aerospace medicine; ammeter; ampicillin; amplitude modulation; anovular menstruation; *ante meridiem* (L) before noon, in the morning; antibodies

to cardiac myosin; arousal mechanism; *Artium Magister* (L) Master of Arts; aviation medicine; axiomesial; meter-angle

Am American; amyl

am ametropia; metre-angle; myopic astigmatism

AMA against medical advice; American Medical Association; antimitochondrial antibodies; Australian Medical Association

AMA-DE American Medical Association Drug Evaluation

AMAL Aeronautical-Medical Acceleration Laboratory

AMB amphotericin B

amb ambulance; ambulatory

ambig ambiguous

ambul ambulation, ambulatory

AMC Animal Medical Center; antimalaria campaign; Army Medical Center; Army Medical Corps; arthrogryposis multiplex congenita; axiomesiocervical

AMD aeromedical data; axiomesiodistal; Aerospace Medical Division (Air Force); Army Medical Department; Association for Macular Diseases

AMDS Association of Military Dental Surgeons

AMEDS Army Medical Service

AMEL Aero-Medical Equipment Laboratory

Amer American

AMF antimuscle factor

AMG amyloglucosidase (glucoamylase); axiomesiogingival

AMH automated medical history

Amh mixed astigmatism with myopia predominating

AMHA Association of Mental Health Administrators

AMI acute myocardial infarction; American Medical International Inc.; amitriptyline hydrochloride; Association of Medical Illustrators; axiomesioincisal

AMIIA Army Medical Intelligence and Information Agency

AML acute myeloblastic leukaemia; anterior mitral leaflet

AMLR autologous mixed lymphocyte reaction

AMM antibodies to murine cardiac myosin; Association Médicale Mondiale (World Medical Association)

AMML acute myelomonocytic leukaemia

AMMOL acute myelomonoblastic leukaemia

ammon ammonia

AMN alloxazine mononucleotide

AMO Assistant Medical Officer; Aviation Medical Officer; axiomesio-occlusal

AMOL acute monoblastic leukaemia

amor amorphous

AMP adenosine monophosphate; amphetamine; average mean pressure

amp ampere, amperage; amplification; ampoule; amputation

AMPA American Medical Publishers Association

amph amphoric

AMPIM Animal Models of Protecting Ischaemic Myocardium

ampl *amplus* (L) large

AMPS acid mucopolysaccharide

ampul *ampulla* (L) ampul, ampoule

AMQ American Medical Qualification (Brit)

AMR activity metabolic rate; alternating motion reflexes; Aviation Medical Reports

AMRL Aerospace Medical Research Laboratories; Army Medical Research and Nutrition Laboratory

AMS abortus, melitensis, suis; acute mountain sickness; American Microscopical Society; Army Medical Service (Brit); Association of Military Surgeons; atypical measles syndrome; auditory memory span; automicrobic system

AMSA acridinylamine methanesulphon-m-anisidide; American Medical Society on Alcoholism; American Medical Students Association; amsacrine

AMSC Army Medical Specialist Corps

AMSRDC Army Medical Service Research and Development Command

AMT American Medical Technologists; amphetamines

amt amount

AMU Army Medical Unit

amu atomic mass unit

AN aneurysm; anisometropia; anode; anodal; anorexia nervosa; antenatal; aseptic necrosis

A/N as needed

A$_n$ normal atmosphere

ANA American Narcolepsy Association; American Neurological Association; American Nurses' Association; anaesthesia, anaesthetic; antinuclear antibody

ANAD anorexia nervosa and associated disorders

Anaes[th] anaesthesia, anaesthetic

anal analgesic; analysis, analyses

ANAP agglutination negative, absorption positive
Anat anatomy(-tomical)
ANC Army Nurse Corps
AnCC anodal closure contraction
ANDRO androsterone
AnDTe anodal duration tetanus
Anesth anesthesia, anesthetic
an ex anode excitation
ANF American Nurses' Foundation; antinuclear factors
Ang angiogram; angle, especially angle of scapula
anh anhydrous
ANIT alpha-naphthyl-isothiocyanate
ANL acute nonlymphoblastic leukaemia
ANLI antibody-negative mice with latent infection
ANLL acute nonlymphocytic leukaemia
Ann annals; annual
Annls annals
AnOC anodal opening contraction
ANP A-norprogesterone
ANRL antihypertensive neutral renomedullary lipids
ANS American Nutrition Society; Army Nursing Service;
　　Associate in Nursing Science; autonomic nervous sys-
　　tem
ans answer
ANSI American National Standards Institute (formerly
　　ASA, USASI)
ANT acoustic noise test; aminonitrothiazole
ant anterior; antimycin
Ant A antimycin A
antag antagonistic
ant ax line anterior axillary line
ante *ante* (L) before
Anthrop anthropology
ant jentac *ante jentaculum* (L) before breakfast
Ant pit anterior pituitary (anterior lobe of pituitary)
Ant sup spine anterior superior spine (of ilium)
ANTU alphanaphthylthiourea
ANUG acute necrotizing ulcerative gingivitis
AO acid output; acridine orange (test); anodal opening;
　　atomic orbital (contour); axio-occlusal
A-O acoustic-optic
AOA American Optometric Association; American
　　Orthopedic Association; American Orthopsychiatric
　　Association; American Osteopathic Association
AOAA amino-oxyacetic acid

AOAC Association of Official Agricultural Chemists
AOAS American Osteopathic Academy of Sclerotherapy
AOB accessory olfactory bulb; alcohol on breath
AOC American Ophthalmological Color Chart; anodal opening contraction
AOCA American Osteopathic College of Anesthesiologists
AOCD American Osteopathic College of Dermatology
AOCI anodal opening clonus
AOCPA American Osteopathic College of Pathologists
AOCPR American Osteopathic College of Proctology
AOCR American Osteopathic College of Radiology; American Osteopathic College of Rheumatology
AOCRM American Osteopathic College of Rehabilitation
AOD Academy of Operative Dentistry; adult onset diabetes; arterial occlusive disease; auriculo-osteodysplasia
AODM adult onset diabetes mellitus
AODME Academy of Osteopathic Directors of Medical Education
AOHA American Osteopathic Hospital Association
AOL acro-osteolysis
AOM Master of Obstetric Art
AOMA American Occupational Medical Association
AOO anodal opening odour
AOP anodal opening picture
AOPA American Orthotic and Prosthetics Association
Aort regurg aortic regurgitation
Aort sten aortic stenosis
AOS American Ophthalmological Society; American Orthodontic Society; American Otological Society; anodal opening sound
AOSSM American Orthopedic Society for Sports Medicine
AOT Association of Occupational Therapists; anti-ovotransferrin
AOTA American Occupational Therapy Association
AOTe anodal opening tetanus
AOU apparent oxygen utilization
AP action potential; alkaline phosphatase; alum precipitated (with reference to vaccines); American Pharmacopeia; angina pectoris; anterior pituitary; anteroposterior; aortic pressure; appendectomy; arithmetic progression; artificial pneumothorax; as prescribed; atrium pace; axiopulpal

A&P auscultation and percussion
AP apothecary
ap *ante prandium* (L) before dinner
A₂>P₂ aortic second sound greater than pulmonary second sound
A₂<P₂ aortic second sound less than pulmonary second sound
APA Administrative Professional Association; American Pancreatic Association; American Pharmaceutical Association; American Physiotherapy Association; American Podiatry Association; American Psychiatric Association; American Psychoanalytic Association; American Psychological Assocation; American Psychopathological Association; American Psychotherapy Association; aminopenicillanic acid
APAF antipernicious anaemia factor
APB atrial premature beats
APC adenoidal, pharyngeal, conjunctival (virus); antigen presenting cell; antiphlogistic corticoid; aperture current; apneustic centre (of brain); aspirin, phenacetin, and caffeine; atrial premature contractions
APCF acute pharyngoconjunctival fever
APCG apex cardiogram
APD action potential duration
A-PD anteroposterior diameter
APE acetone powder extract; anterior pituitary extract
APF acidulated phosphofluoride; American Psychological Foundation; animal protein factor
APG acid-precipitable globulin
APGAR American Pediatric Gross Assessment Record
APH anterior pituitary hormone; Association of Private Hospitals
APHA American Protestant Hospital Association; American Public Health Association
APhA American Pharmaceutical Association
API Analytical Profile Index (microbiology)
APIC Association for Practitioners in Infection Control
APIM Association Professionelle Internationale des Médecins
APIP additional personal injury protection
APKD adult-onset polycystic kidney disease
APL acute promyelocytic leukaemia; anterior-pituitary-like substance
AP&Lat anteroposterior and lateral

APM Academy of Parapsychology and Medicine; Academy of Physical Medicine; Academy of Psychosomatic Medicine; acid-precipitable material; aspartame; Association of Professors of Medicine

APMR Association for Physical and Mental Rehabilitation

APO apomorphine

apoth apothecary

APP alum-precipitated protein; avian pancreatic polypeptide

app apparent; appendix

APPA American Psychopathological Association

appar apparatus; apparent

APPG aqueous procaine penicillin G

appl appliance; applied

applan *applanatus* (L) flattened

applicand *applicandus* (L) to be applied

appr approximate(ly)

approx approximate(ly)

appt appointment

Appx appendix

aprax apraxia

APRL American Prosthetic Research Laboratory

AProL acute progranulocytic leukaemia

APS adenosine phosphosulphate; American Pediatric Society; American Physiological Society; American Proctologic Society; American Prosthodontic Society; American Psychological Society; American Psychosomatic Society

APSS Association for Psychophysiological Study of Sleep

APT alum-precipitated toxoid

APTA American Physical Therapy Association

APTC Army Physical Training Corps

APTD Aid to Permanently and Totally Disabled

APTT activated partial thromboplastin time

APUD amine precursor uptake and decarboxylation (cells)

AQ accomplishment or achievement quotient; any quantity

aq *aqua* (L) water; aqueous

aq astr *aqua astricta* (L) frozen water

aq bull *aqua bulliens* (L) boiling water

aq cal *aqua calida* (L) hot water

aq comm *aqua communis* (L) common water

aq dest *aqua destillata* (L) distilled water

aq ferv *aqua fervens* (L) hot water
aq fluv *aqua fluvialis* (L) river water
aq font *aqua fontana* (L) spring water
aq frig *aqua frigada* (L) cold water
aq mar *aqua marina* (L) sea water
aq niv *aqua nivalis* (L) snow water
aq pluv *aqua pluvialis* (L) rain water
aq pur *aqua pura* (L) pure water
aq tep *aqua tepida* (L) lukewarm water
aqu aqueous
AR achievement ratio; active resistance (exercise); alarm reaction; allergic rhinitis; analytical reagent; androgen receptor; aortic regurgitation; apical-radial (pulse) arsphenamine; articulare (craniometric point); artificial respiration; atrophic rhinitis (of swine); autoradiography
A/R apical/radial
Ar argon
ARA Academy of Rehabilitative Audiometry; American Rheumatism Association; Associate of the Royal Academy
ara-A adenine arabinoside (vidarabine)
ara-C cytosine arabinoside (cytarabine)
ARBOR arthropod-borne (virus)
ARC accelerating rate calorimeter; Addiction Research Center (NIMH); American Red Cross; anomalous retinal correspondence; arcuate nucleus (of the brain); Arthritis Rehabilitation Center; Association for Retarded Children
ARCA acquired red cell aplasia
Arch archives
ARCI Addiction Research Center Inventory
ARCS Associate of the Royal College of Science
ARD absolute reaction of degeneration; acute respiratory disease; arthritis and rheumatic diseases
ARDC Air Research and Development Command
ARDS acute respiratory distress syndrome
ARF acute rheumatic fever; Addiction Research Foundation
Arg arginine
arg *argentum* (L) silver
ARI airway reactivity index
ARIA automated radioimmunoassay
ARM allergy relief medicine; artificial rupture of the

membranes; atomic resolution microscope
ARN   Association of Rehabilitation Nurses
ARNMD   Association for Research in Nervous and Mental Diseases
ARNP   Advanced Registered Nurse Practitioner
ARO   Associate for Research in Ophthalmology
ARP   absolute refractory period; Advanced Research Projects; American Registry of Pathologists
ARPT   American Registry of Physical Therapists
ARRC   Associate of the Royal Red Cross
ARRS   American Roentgen Ray Society
ARRT   American Registered Respiratory Therapist
ARS   alizarin red S; American Radium Society; American Rhinologic Society; antirabies serum
Ars   arsphenamine
ARSA   American Reye's Syndrome Association
ARSC   Associate of the Royal Society of Chemistry
ARSM   acute respiratory system malfunction
ARSPH   Associate of the Royal Society for the Promotion of Health
ART   Accredited Record Technician; acoustic reflex test
art   artery, arterial; articulation; artificial
artic   articulation
artif   artificial
art insem   artificial insemination
AS   active sleep; alimentary sleep; ankylosing spondylitis; antiserum; anxiety state; aortic stenosis; aqueous solution; aqueous suspension; arteriosclerosis; artificial sweetener; asymmetric; audiogenic seizure; *auris sinistra* (L) left ear
A-S   ascendance-submission
As   arsenic; astigmatism
ASA   acetylsalicylic acid (aspirin); American Society of Anesthesiologists; American Standards Association
ASAIO   American Society for Artificial Internal Organs
ASAP   American Society for Adolescent Psychology; as soon as possible
ASB   American Society of Bacteriology
ASC   acetylsulphanilyl chloride
asc   arteriosclerosis(-sclerotic); ascending
ASCH   American Society of Clinical Hypnosis
ASCLT   American Society of Clinical Laboratory Technicians
ASCMS   American Society of Contemporary Medicine and Surgery

ASCO American Society of Clinical Oncology; American Society of Contemporary Ophthalmology

ASCP American Society of Clinical Pathologists; American Society of Consulting Pharmacists

ASCR American Society of Chiropodical Roentgenology

ascr *ascriptum* (L) ascribed to

ASCVD arteriosclerotic cardiovascular disease

ASD atrial septal defect

ASDA American Society for Dental Aesthetics; American Student Dental Association

ASDC American Society of Dentistry for Children; Association of Sleep Disorders Centers

ASDH acute subdural haematoma

ASDR American Society of Dental Radiographers

ASE axilla, shoulder, elbow (bandage)

ASF alinine, sulphur, and formaldehyde (microscopy)

ASG American Society for Genetics; Army Surgeon General

ASGB Anatomical Society of Great Britain and Ireland

ASGD American Society for Geriatric Dentistry

ASGE American Society for Gastrointestinal Endoscopy

ASH American Society for Hematology; asymmetric septal hypertrophy

AsH hypermetropic astigmatism

ASHA American School Health Association; American Social Health Association; American Speech and Hearing Association

ASHBM Associate Scottish Hospital Bureau of Management

ASHD arteriosclerotic heart disease

ASHG American Society for Human Genetics

ASHI Association for Study of Human Infertility

ASHNS American Society for Head and Neck Surgery

ASHP American Society of Hospital Pharmacists; American Society for Hospital Planning

ASHPA American Society for Hospital Personnel Administration

ASII American Science Information Institute

ASIM American Society of Internal Medicine

ASL antistreptolysin titre

ASLIB Association of Special Libraries and Information Bureaux

ASLM American Society of Law and Medicine

ASLO antistreptolysin-O

ASM American Society for Microbiology

AsM myopic astigmatism
ASME Association for the Study of Medical Education
ASMPA Armed Services Medical Procurement Agency
ASMR age-standardized mortality ratio
ASMT American Society of Medical Technology
ASN American Society of Nephrology; American Society for Neurochemistry; Associate in Nursing
Asn asparagine
ASO American Society of Orthodontists; antistreptolysin-O; arteriosclerosis obliterans
ASOS American Society of Oral Surgeons
ASP American Society of Parasitologists; American Society of Periodontists (now AAP)
Asp aspartic acid
ASPA American Society of Physician Analysts; American Society of Podiatric Assistants
ASPM American Society of Paramedics
ASPO American Society for Psychoprophylaxis in Obstetrics
ASPP Association for Sane Psychiatric Practices
ASR aldosterone secretion rate
ASRT American Society of Radiologic Technologists
ASS anterior superior spine
Assn association
Assoc associate, association
assocd associated (with)
asst assistant
AST angiotensin sensitivity test; aspartate aminotransferase; Association of Medical Technologists; audiometry sweep test (Brit)
Ast astigmatism
ASTA anti-alpha-staphylolysin
ASTEC Association of Science Technology Centers
A sten aortic stenosis
Asth asthenopia
ASTHO Association of State and Territorial Health Officials
ASTI antispasticity index
ASTM American Society for Testing and Materials
ASTMH American Society of Tropical Medicine and Hygiene
ASTO antistreptolysin-O
ASTZ antistreptozyme
As tol as tolerated
ASU Aeromedical Staging Unit

A/SV arterio/superficial venous

ASVO American Society of Veterinary Ophthalmology

ASVPP American Society of Veterinary Physiologists and Pharmacologists

asym asymmetrical

AT achievement test; Achilles tendon; adenine and thymine; adjunctive therapy; air temperature; *alt Tuberculin* (Ger) old tuberculin; aminotransferase; amitriptyline; anaphylatoxin; antithrombin; ataxia telangiectasia; attenuated(-uation)

AT₇ hexachlorophane

AT₁₀ dihydrotachysterol

at airtight; atom(ic)

ATA alimentary toxic aleukia; American Thyroid Association; American Tinnitus Association; antithyroglobulin antibody

ATC activated thymus cells

ATCC American Type Culture Collection

ATD Alzheimer type dementia; androstatrienedione; anthropomorphic test dummy

ATDC Association of Thalidomide Damaged Children

at fib atrial fibrillation

ATG adenine, thymine, guanine; antihuman thymocyte globulin; antithrombocyte globulin

ATGAM antithymocyte gamma globulin

ATH acetyl-tyrosine hydrazide

ATh Associate in Therapy

ATHC allotetrahydrocortisol

Athsc atherosclerosis

ATL Achilles tendon lengthening; adult T-cell leukaemia

ATLA adult T-cell leukaemia antigen

ATLS Advanced Trauma Life Support Program

ATLV adult T-cell leukaemia virus

atm atmosphere(-spheric)

atmos atmosphere(-spheric)

ATN acute tubular necrosis

at no atomic number

ATP adenosine triphosphate

ATPase adenosine triphosphatase

ATPD ambient temperature and pressure, dry

ATPS ambient temperature and pressure, saturated

ATR Achilles tendon reflex

atr atrophy

ATS American Therapeutic Society (now ASCPT); American Thoracic Society; American Trudeau

Society; American Trauma Society; antitetanus serum; anxiety tension state

att attending

at wt atomic weight

AU *ad usum* (L) according to custom; Ångström unit; antitoxin unit (diphtheria); *aures unitas* (L) both ears (together); *auris uterque* (L) each ear; Australia (antigen)

Au gold (L) *aurum*

¹⁹⁸Au radioactive gold

AUA American Urological Association; Association of University Anesthetists

auct *auctorum* (L) of authors

aud auditory

aug *augere* (L) increase

AUL acute undifferentiated leukaemia

AUO amyloid of unknown origin

aur *auris* (L) ear; *aurum* (L) gold

aur fib auricular fibrillation

auric auricular

aurin *aurinarium* (L) ear cone

aurist *auristillae* (L) ear drops

AuSH Australian serum hepatitis

aux auxiliary

AV anterior-ventral; anteversion(-verted); aortic valve; arteriovenous; atrioventricular; auriculoventricular; average; avoirdupois

AVA arteriovenous anastomosis

AVC Academy of Veterinary Cardiology; allantoid vaginal cream; atrioventricular canal; Association of Vitamin Chemists; associative visual cortex

AVD Army Veterinary Department (Brit)

avdp avoirdupois

AVE aortic valve echocardiogram

AVF antiviral factor

avg average

AVI air velocity index; Association of Veterinary Inspectors;

Aviat Med Aviation Medicine

AVM arteriovenous malfunction; Aviation Medicine

AVMA American Veterinary Medical Association

AVN atrioventricular node

AVP antiviral protein; arginine vasopressin

AVS Association for Voluntary Sterilization

AVT arginine vasotocin; area ventralis of Tsai (of the

brain); Aviation Medicine Technician
AW above waist; atomic warfare
A/W in accordance with
A & W alive and well
AWF adrenal weight factor
AWP airway pressure
AWRS anti-whole rabbit serum
ax axillary; axis; axial
AXAF Advanced X-ray Astrophysics Facility
AXF Advanced X-ray Facility
ax grad axial gradient
AXM acetoxycyclo-hexamine
AXT alternating exotropia
AYF antiyeast factor
AYP autolysed yeast protein
Az azote (nitrogen)
AZT Aschheim-Zondek test

B

B *Bacillus; balneum* (L) bath; barometric; base (in chemical formulas); base (of prism); bath; Baumé scale;
behaviour; bel; Benoist scale; benzoate; beta; bicuspid;
blue; body (in psychology, all the body except nervous
system); bone-marrow derived (lymphocytes); boron;
bound; brother; buccal; bursa cells (of thymus or lymph
nodes)
b *bis* (L) twice, two times; boils at (when followed by a
figure designating degrees); born
β beta; In organic compounds, refers to the carbon atom
next but one to the carbon atom bearing the active
group of molecules; Symbol designating *second*
BA Bachelor of Arts; backache; *balneum arenae* (L) sand
bath; basion (craniometric point); benzyladenine;
blood agar; boric acid; breathing apparatus; bronchial
asthma; buccoaxial
B>A bone greater than air (conduction)
Ba barium
BAA benzoyl arginine amide; branched-chain amino acid
BAB blood agar base
Bab Babinski (reflex)
BAC bacterial adherent colonies; bacterial antigen com-
plex; blood alcohol concentration; British Association
of Chemists; bronchoalveolar cells; buccoaxiocervical

Bact *Bacterium*
bact bacteria(l); bacteriology
BAD biological aerosol detection; British Association of Dermatologists
BaE barium enema
Ba enem barium enema
BAEP brainstem auditory evoked potential
BAG buccoaxiogingival
BAGG buffered azide glucose glycerol (broth)
BAL blood alcohol level; British anti-lewisite (dimercaprol); bronchoalveolar lavage
bal balance(d); balsam
bal arenae *balneum arenae* (L) sand bath
B-ALL B-cell acute lymphoblastic leukaemia
bal mar *balneum maris* (L) salt or sea-water bath
bal vap *balneum vapour* (L) steam or vapour bath
bals *balsamum* (L) balsam
BaM barium meal
BAN British Association of Neurologists
BAO Bachelor of the Art of Obstetrics; basal acid output; British Association of Otolaryngologists
BAP blood agar plate; bovine albumin in phosphate buffer; brachial artery pressure
BAPhysMed British Association of Physical Medicine
BAPN beta-amino-proprionitrile fumarate
BAPS British Association of Paediatric Surgeons; British Association of Plastic Surgeons
BAPT British Association of Physical Training
bar barometer; barometric
BAS benzyl analogue of serotonin; Bioanalytical Systems
bas basophil(s)
BASH body acceleration synchronous with heart beat
basos basophils
BAT brown adipose tissue
BAUS British Association of Urological Surgeons
BAW bronchoalveolar wash fluids
BB bad breath; bed bath; beta-blocker; blanket bath; blood bank; both bones (with reference to fractures); breakthrough bleeding; breast biopsy
BBA born before arrival
BBB blood-brain barrier; bundle-branch block
BBC brombenzylcyanide
BBE bacteroides bile esculin (agar)
BBS bombesin
BBT basal body temperature

BB/W Biobreeding/Worcester (rats)

BC *Baccalaureus Chirurgiae* (L); Bachelor of Surgery; bipolar cell; birth control; Blue Cross; bone conduction; bronchial carcinoma; buccal cartilage; buccocervical

BCA Blue Cross Association

BCB brilliant cresyl blue

BC/BS Blue Cross/Blue Shield

BCC basal cell carcinoma; Birth Control Clinic

BCCG British Co-operative Clinical Group

BCCP biotin carboxyl carrier protein

BCE basal cell epithelioma

BCF basophil chemotactic factor

BCFP breast cyst fluid protein

BCG bacille Calmette-Guérin; ballistocardiogram; bromcresyl green

BCG test bicolour guaiac test

BCH basal cell hyperplasia

BCh Bachelor of Surgery

BChD Bachelor of Dental Surgery

BChir *Baccalaurens Chirurgiae* (L) Bachelor of Surgery

BChL bacteriochlorophyll

BCIC Birth Control Investigation Committee

B-CLL B-cell chronic lymphatic leukaemia

BCLS Basic Cardiac Life Support System

BCM birth control medication

bcm billion cubic meters

BCME bis-chlormethyl ether

BCNU 1, 3-bis(2-chloroethyl)-1-nitrosourea (carmustine)

BCP Blue Cross Plan; bromcresyl purple

BCS battered child syndrome; blood cell separator; British Cardiac Society

BCTF Breast Cancer Task Force (NCI)

BCSI breast cancer screening indicator

BCV basal cell vigilance

BCW Biological and Chemical Warefare

BD base deficit; base of prism down; Batten's disease; behavioural disorder; belladonna; Best delay (audiometry); bile duct; binocular deprivation; Black Death; borderline dull; bound; buccodistal; bundle

B&D bondage and discipline

Bd board

bd *bis die*(L) twice a day

BDA British Dental Association

BDAC Bureau of Drug Abuse Control

BDB bis-diazotized-benzidine
BDC burn-dressing change
BDE bile duct examination
BDentSci Bachelor of Dental Science (Dublin)
BDG buffered desoxycholate glucose (broth)
BDH British Drug Houses Ltd.
BDI Becton Dickinson Diagnostics
BDL below detectable limits; bundle
BDS Bachelor of Dental Surgery; biological detection system
bds *bis in die summendus* (L) to be taken twice a day
BDSc Bachelor of Dental Science
BDU Biomedical Display Unit
BDUR bromodeoxyuridine
BE Bacillary Emulsion; barium enema; base excess; below elbow; bile esculin; breast examination; broncho-esophagology
Be beryllium
Bé Beaumé (specific gravity scale)
BEAM brain electrical activity map
BEAR Biological Effects of Atomic Radiation (Committee)
beg begin
beh behaviour(ism)
BEI butanol-extractable iodine
ben *bene* (L) well, good
Benz benzidine
BEP brain evoked potential
BER basic electrical rhythm
BES balanced electrolyte solution
BESS Biomedical Experimental Scientific Satellite
bet between
BEV baboon endogenous virus
beV billion electron volts
BF bentonite flocculation (test); blastogenic factor; *bouillon filtre* (Fr) bouillon filtrate tuberculin; Denys' tuberculin; breakfast fed; buffered; butter fat
B/F bound/free (antigens)
BFB biological feedback
BFL bird-fancier's lung
BFP biological false positive
BFR sol buffered Ringer's solution
BFV bovine faeces virus
BG bicolour guaiac (test); blood glucose; brilliant green; buccogingival

B-G Bordet-Gengou (bacillus)
BGC blood group class
BGE butyl glycidyl ether
BGG bovine gamma globulin
BGGRA British Gelatine and Glue Research Association
BGLB brilliant green lactose broth
BGS blood group substance; British Geriatrics Society
BH Base Hospital; bill of health; Board of Health; brain hormone
BHAT betablocker heart attack trial
BHC benzene hexachloride
BHI biosynthetic human insulin; brain-heart infusion; Bureau of Health Insurance
BHI-ac brain-heart infusion broth with acetone
BHIB beef heart infusion broth
BHIBA brain-heart infusion blood agar
BHIS beef heart infusion supplemented (broth or agar)
BHL biological half-life
BHM Bureau of Health Manpower
BHN bephenium hydroxynaphthoate
BHP Basic Health Profile
BHPRD Bureau of Health Planning and Resources Development
BHR basal heart rate
BHS Bachelor of Health Science
BHT beta-hydroxytheophylline; breath hydrogen test
BHyg Bachelor of Hygiene
BI base of prism in; biological indicator; bodily injury; bone injury; Braille Institute
Bi bismuth
BIAC Beth Israel Ambulatory Center; Bioinstrumentation Advisory Council
bib *bibe* (L) drink
biblio bibliography
BIBRA British Industrial Biological Research Association
BIC Biomedical Instrumentation Consultant
bicarb bicarbonate
BiCNU BCNU
BID brought in dead
bid *bis in die* (L) twice a day
BIGGY bismuth glycine glucose yeast (agar)
BIH benign intracranial hypertension
bihor *bihorium* (L) during two hours

Bi Isch between ischial tuberosities
BIL bilirubin (test)
bilat bilateral
bili, bilirub bilirubin
bin *bis in noctus* (L) twice a night
BioAb Biological Abstracts
Biochem biochemistry(-ical)
Biol biology(-ological)
Biophys biophysics
BIP bacterial intravenous protein; biparietal diameter (of skull); bismuth iodoform paraffin; Blue Cross Interim Payment
BIPM *Bureau International des Poids et Mesures* (International Bureau of Weights and Measures)
BIPP bismuth iodoform paraffin paste
BIR basic incidence rate; British Institute of Radiology
BiSP between ischial spines
BiT between great trochanters
BJ Bence Jones (protein); biceps jerk
B&J bone and joint
BJM bones, joints, muscles
BK below knee (with reference to amputation stump)
BKA below the knee amputation
bkf breakfast
BKTT below knee to toe
BKWP below knee walking plaster
BL black light; bone marrow derived lymphocyte; buccolingual; Burkitt's lymphoma
Bl black
bl bleeding; blood; blue
B-l bursa equivalent lymphocyte
BLAD borderline left axis deviation
BLB mask Boothby-Lovelace-Bulbulian mask
BlC blood culture
bl cult blood culture
BLG beta-lactoglobulin
BLM bimolecular liquid membrane
BLOT British Library of Tape (Recordings)
BlP blood pressure
BLROA British Laryngological, Rhinological and Otological Association
BLS Basic Life Support Systems; blood and lymphatic systems
BlS blood sugar
BlT blood type

BLV bovine leukaemia virus

BM Bachelor of Medicine; basal medium; basal metabolism; basilar membrane; blind matching (parapsychology); bowel movement; buccal mass (dentistry); buccomesial; Bureau of Medicine

bm *balneum maris* (L) sea-water bath

BMA British Medical Association

BMB biomedical belt

BME basal medium, Eagle's

BMed Bachelor of Medicine

BMedBiol Bachelor of Medical Biology

BMedSci Bachelor of Medical Science

BMic Bachelor of Microbiology

B-mod behaviour modification

BMP bone morphogenic protein

BMPP benign mucous membrane pemphigus

BMQA Board of Medical Quality Assurance

BMR basal metabolic rate

BMS Bachelor of Medical Science; Biomedical Monitoring System; bleomycin sulphate; Bureau of Medicine and Surgery (Navy)

BMSA British Medical Students Association

BMT Baillière's Medical Transparencies; Bachelor of Medical Technology; bone marrow transplant

BNA Basle (Basel) Nomina Anatomica

BNDD Bureau of Narcotics and Dangerous Drugs

BNEd Bachelor of Nursing Education

BNF British National Formulary

BNO bowels not opened

BNSc Bachelor of Nursing Science

BO Bachelor of Osteopathy; base of prism out; body odour; Bolton (craniometric point); bowels open; bucco-occlusal

bo bowel

B&O belladonna and opium

BOA born on arrival; British Orthopaedic Association

BOD biochemical oxygen demand; biological oxygen demand

BodUnit Bodansky unit

BOEA ethyl biscoumacetate

BOH Board of Health

boil boiling

bol *bolus* (L) a large pill

BONENT Board of Nephrology Examiners for Nursing and Technology

BOP Buffalo orphan prototype (with reference to viruses)

BOR bowels open regularly

Bot botany, botanical

bot bottle

BOW bag of waters (amniotic sac)

BP Bachelor of Pharmacy; barometric pressure; basic protein; bathroom privileges; bed pan; biotic potential; biparietal (diameter of head); birth place; blood pressure; British Pharmacopoeia; buccopulpal; bypass

bp base pairs (of DNA); boiling point

BPA blood pressure assembly; bovine plasma albumin; British Paediatric Association

BPB bromophenol blue

BPC British Pharmaceutical Codex

BPD biparietal diameter; Blood Program Directives (Red Cross); bronchopulmonary dysplasia

BPE bacterial phosphatidylethanolamine

BPF burst-promoting factor

BPG blood pressure gauge

BPH Bachelor of Public Health; benign prostatic hypertrophy

BPharm Bachelor of Pharmacy

BPHEng Bachelor of Public Health Engineering

BPheo bacteriopheophytin

BPHN Bachelor of Public Health Nursing

BPL β-propriolactone

BP 120/80 lar blood pressure 120 (systolic), 80 (diastolic), left arm reclining or recumbent

BPM brompheniramine maleate

BPMF British Postgraduate Medical Federation

BPMS blood plasma measuring system

BPP bovine pancreatic polypeptide

BPR blood pressure recorder

BPRS Brief Psychiatric Rating Scale

BPS beats per second; Behavioral Pharmacological Society; Biophysical Society; brain protein solvent; breaths per second

BPsTh Bachelor of Psychotherapy

BPV bovine papilloma virus

BP(Vet) British Pharmacopoeia (veterinary)

BQC Dibromoquinone-chlorimide

Bq becquerel (SI)

BR bathroom; bed rest; British Revision of BNA (with reference to anatomical nomenclature)

Br bridge (dentistry); British; bromine; bronchitis; brown; *Brucella*

br boiling range; branch; breath; brother

BRBA *Brucella,* vitamin K blood agar

BRBNS blue rubber-bleb naevus syndrome

BRCS British Red Cross Society

BrDU bromodeoxyuridine

BrdUrd bromodeoxyuridine

Brhp bronchophony

BRI Bio-Research Index

Brit British

Brkf breakfast

BRL Beecham Research Laboratories; Bethesda Research Laboratories; Biometrics Research Laboratory

BRN Board of Registered Nursing

BRO bronchoscopy

Bron bronchial

Bronch bronchoscopy(-scopist)

BRP bathroom privileges

BRS British Roentgen Society

BS Bachelor of Science; Bachelor of Surgery; bismuth subsalicylate; blood sugar; Bloom syndrome; Blue Shield; bowel sound; breath sound; British Standard; Bureau of Standards

B&S Bartholin's and Skene's (glands)

BSA benzenesulphonic acid; Biofeedback Society of America; Blind Service Association; Blue Shield Association; body surface area; bovine serum albumin

BSC Bench scale calorimeter; Biological Stain Commission; Biomedical Sciences Corps (Air Force); Biomedical Signal Conditioner

BSc Bachelor of Science

BSCC British Society for Clinical Cytology

BSE breast self-examination

BSI British Standards Institution

BSL benign symmetric lipomatoses; blood sugar level

BSM Bachelor of Science in Medicine

BSN Bachelor of Science in Nursing; bowel sounds normal

BSO bilateral salpingo-oophorectomy; British School of Osteopathy

BSOT Bachelor of Science in Occupational Therapy

BSP Bromsulphalein

BSp bronchospasm

BSPh Bachelor of Science in Pharmacy

BSR blood sedimentation rate; brain stimulation reinforcement

BSS Bachelor of Sanitary Science; buffered salt (saline) solution

BST blood serological test; brief stimulus therapy (psychology)

BT *Bacillus thuringiensis;* bedtime; bitemporal (diameter of head); blue tetrazolium; body temperature; brain tumour

BTA Blood Transfusion Association

BTB breakthrough bleeding; bromthymol blue

BTH butylated hydroxytolulene

BThU British Thermal Unit

BTMD Batten-Turner Muscular Dystrophy

BTPS body temperature, pressure (prevailing atmospheric), and saturation (water vapour)

BTS Blood Transfusion Service

BTSG Brain Tumor Study Group (National Cancer Institute)

BTU British Thermal Unit

BTX benzene, toluene, xylene; bungarotoxin

BTX-B brevetoxin-B

BU base of prism up; Bodansky unit; bromouracil; Burn Unit

Bu butyl

Buc buccal

BUDU bromodeoxyuridine

BUG buccal ganglion

BUI brain uptake index

bull bulletin; *bulliat* (L) let it boil

BuMed Bureau of Medicine and Surgery, US Navy

BUN blood urea nitrogen

BUO bleeding or bruising of undetermined origin

BUPA British United Provident Association

Bur buried

bur bureau

Burd Burdick suction

BUS busulphan

But *butyrum* (L) butter

BUTE phenylbutazone

BV bacitracin V; biological value; blood vessel; blood volume

bv *balneum vaporis* (L) vapour bath

BVA Blinded Veterans Association; British Veterinary Association

BVDT Brief Vestibular Disorientation Test
BVE binocular visual efficiency
BVM bronchovascular markings; Bureau of Veterinary Medicine
BVMS Bachelor of Veterinary Medicine and Surgery
BVP blood vessel prosthesis
BVSc Bachelor of Veterinary Science
BVU bromoisovalerylurea
BVX bacitracin V and X
BW bacteriological warfare; below waist; biological warfare; biological weapons; birth weight; bladder washout; blood Wassermann; body water; body weight
BWD bacillary white diarrhoea (in chicks)
BWRWS Biological Warfare Rapid Warning System
BWSV black widow spider venom
BWt birth weight
BX bacitracin X; biopsy
BYE Barile-Yaguchi-Eveland (medium)
BZ benzodiazepine; benzoyl

C

C A symbol for any constant; Caesarean section; calorie (large); canine tooth (permanent); carbohydrate; carbon; carrier; cathode; Roman Catholic; Celsius scale or thermometer; centigrade (temperature scale); central; certified; cervical; chest (precordial) lead; chloramphenicol; clearance (renal); clonus; closure; coarse (with reference to bacterial colonies); cocaine; coefficient; coloured; colour sense; complement; complete; compliance; component; *compositus* (L) compound; concentration; conditioning(-tioned); *congius* (L) gallon; consultation; contraction; control (with reference to a group in an experiment); *contusus* (L) bruised; cortex; costa (rib); coulomb (SI); Coxsackie (virus); crystalline enzyme; cylinder; cytidine; cytochrome; cytosine
c calorie (small); candle; canine tooth (deciduous); capacity; centi (prefix); *centum* (L) one hundred; *cibus* (L) meal; *circa* (L) about; contact; cubic; *cum* (L) with; curie; cyclic
c̄ with
C' complement (bacteriology)

C1, C2, C3 (etc) cervical nerves or cervical vertebrae No. 1, No. 2, No. 3 (etc)

CI, CII, CIII (etc) cranial nerves I, II, etc

C_1, C_2, C_3 costa (rib) I (first rib), etc; cytochromes 1, 2 and 3

C_1 to C_9 components of complement

C_3 Collin's solution (for perfusion)

C10 decamethonium iodide

^{14}C radioactive carbon

C_{alb} albumin clearance

C_{cr} creatinine clearance

C_{in} inulin clearance

C_p phosphate clearance

C_{pah} p-aminohippurate clearance

C_{T-1824} clearance of Evans blue

CA carbonic anhydrase; carcinoma; cardiac arrest; catecholamine; cerebral aqueduct; cervicoaxial; Chemical Abstracts; chronological age; coagglutination (test); coeliac axis; colloid antigen; commissural-association (zone of the brain); common antigen; coronary artery; corpora alata; corpora amylacea; cortisone acetate; Council Accepted (American Medical Association); croup-associated (virus); cytosine arabinoside

Ca calcium; carcinoma; cathode, cathodal

ca candle; *circa* (L) about (with reference to time)

CAA constitutional aplastic anaemia

CAAT computer-assisted axial tomography

CAB coronary artery bypass

CABG coronary artery bypass graft

CABGS coronary artery bypass graft surgery

CABP calcium-binding protein

CAC cardiac-accelerator centre; cardiac arrest code

CaCC cathodal closure contraction

CACX cancer of the cervix

CAD computer-assisted diagnosis; coronary artery disease

Cad cadaver

CaDTe cathodal duration tetanus

CAE contingent after-effects

CaEDTA calcium disodium ethylenediaminetetra-acetate (edathamil calcium disodium)

caerul *caeruleus* (L) dark blue, dark green

CAF cell adhesion factor; citric acid fermenters; Cooley's Anemia Foundation

caf caffeine

CAG chronic atrophic gastritis

CAH chronic active hepatitis; congenital adrenal hyperplasia; cyanacetic acid hydrazine

CAHEA Committee on Allied Health Education and Accreditation

CAI computer-aided instruction; confused artificial insemination

CAL calcium test (dentistry); calculated average life; chronic airflow limitation

Cal calorie (large)

cal calibre; calorie (small)

calCd calculated

CALD chronic active liver disease

calef *calefactus* (L) warmed; or *calefac* (L) make warm

CALGB Cancer and Leukaemia, Group B

cALL common null cell acute lymphoblastic leukaemia

CALLA common acute lymphoblastic leukaemia antigen

CAM cell-associating molecule; chorio-allantoic membrane

CaM calmodulin

CAMAC computer automated measurement and control

CAMP Christie, Atkins, Munch-Peterson (test)

cAMP cyclic adenosine monophosphate

Can cancer

CA/N child abuse and neglect

canc cancelled

CAO chronic airway obstruction

CaOC cathodal opening contraction

CAP cell-attachment protein; chloramphenicol; College of American Pathologists; Community Action Program; cystine aminopeptidase

cap capacity; *capiat* (L) let him take; *capsula* (L) capsule

CAPD continuous ambulatory peritoneal dialysis

capiend *capiendus* (L) to be taken

cap moli *capsula mollis* (L) soft capsule

cap quant vult *capiat quantum vult* (L) let the patient take as much as he will

CAPRI Cardiopulmonary Research Institute

caps *capsule* (L) capsule

CAR Canadian Association of Radiologists; computer-assisted research; conditioned avoidance response

carb carbonate

carbo carbohydrate

Cardiol cardiology

CARF Commission on Accreditation and Rehabilitation Facilities

CAS cardiac adjustment scale; carotid artery system; Center for Alcohol Studies; Chemical Abstracts Service; Civil Air Surgeon; control adjustment strap; Council of Academic Societies

Cas casualty

CASA Computer-assisted Self Assessment (Brit)

CASHD coronary arteriosclerotic heart disease

CAS-REGN Chemical Abstracts Service Registry Number

CASS Coronary Artery Surgery Study

CAST Clearinghouse Announcements in Science and Technology

CAT catecholamines; child's apperception test; chloramphenicol acetyltransferase; choline acetyltransferase; classified anaphylatoxin; college ability test; computerized axial tomography

CAT-A-KIT Catecholamines Radioenzymatic Assay Kit

CATCH Community Actions to Control High Blood Pressure (HHS)

Cath Catholic

cath cathartic; catheter(ize)

CATSCAN computerized axial tomography scanner

Cau Caucasian

Caud caudal

CAV congenital absence of vagina; congenital adrenal virilism

cav cavity

CAVD In psychology, a battery of four tests of intelligence (completion, arithmetic problems, vocabulary, following directions)

CB carbenicillin; chest-back; *Chirurgiae Baccalaureus* (L) Bachelor of Surgery; chronic bronchitis

CB$_{11}$ phenadoxine

CBA chronic bronchitis and asthma

CBC complete blood count

CBD closed bladder drainage; common bile duct

CBF cerebral blood flow; cortical blood flow (urology)

CBG corticosteroid-binding globulin (transcortin)

CBI close-binding-intimate

CBL cord (umbilical) blood leucocytes

Cbl cobalamin

CBMMP chronic benign mucous membrane pemphigus

CBN Commission on Biological Nomenclature

CBR chemical, biological and radiological (warefare); complete bed rest; crude birth rate

CBS chronic brain syndrome

CBW chemical, biological warfare; critical band width (of noise)

BCz carbobenzoxychloride

CC calcium cyclamate; cerebral commissure; choriocarcinoma; chief complaint; classical conditioning; clean catch (of urine); closing capacity; coefficient of correlation; commission certified (with reference to stains); compound cathartic; computer calculated; corpora cardiaca; corpus callosum; critical care; critical condition; current complaints

Cc concave

cc cubic centimetre; with correction (ophthalmology)

CCA cephalin cholesterol antigen; chick cell agglutination (unit); chimpanzee coryza agent

C-C-A cytidyl-cytidyl-adenyl

CCAT conglutinating complement absorption test

CCBB Clinical Center Blood Bank

CCBV central circulating blood volume

CCC calcium cyanamide (carbimide) citrated; cathodal closure contraction

CCCC centrifugal countercurrent chromatography

CCCI cathodal closure clonus

CCCR closed chest cardiac resuscitation

CCD calibration curve data

CCDC Canadian Communicable Disease Center

CCDN Central Council for District Nursing

CCE carboline-carboxylic acid ester; clear-cell carcinoma (of the endothelium)

CCF congestive cardiac failure; crystal-induced chemotactic factor

CCFA cefoxitin cycloserine fructose agar medium

CCHE Central Council for Health Education

CCHMS Central Committee for Hospital Medical Services (Brit)

CCHP Consumer Choice Health Plan

CCHS congenital central hypoventilation syndrome

CCI chronic coronary insufficiency

CCK cholecystokinin

CCL carcinoma cell line; critical carbohydrate level

CCME Coordinating Council of Medical Education

CCMS clean catch midstream

CCNS cell cycle nonspecific (antitumour agent)
CCNU 1-(-2-chloroethyl)-3-cyclohexyl-1-nitrosourea
CCP ciliocytopathoria
CCPDS Centralized Cancer Patient Data System
CCRN Critical Care Registered Nurse
CCS casualty clearing station; cell cycle specific (anti-tumour agent); concentration camp syndrome
CCT chocolate-coated tablet; coated compressed tablet; controlled cord traction; Coronary Care Team
CCTe cathodal closure tetanus
CCU Cardiac Care Unit; colour changing units; Coronary Care Unit; Critical Care Unit
CCW counter clockwise
CD cadaver donor; Caesarean delivered; canine distemper; canine dose; cardiovascular disease; Carrel-Dakin (fluid); civil defence; *colla dextra* (L) with the right hand; combination drug; communicable disease; completely denatured; *conjugata diagonalis* (L) diagonal conjugate (diameter of pelvic inlet); contact dermatitis; control diet; convulsive disorder; convulsive dose; Crohn's disease; curative dose; cystic duct
Cd cadmium; caudal or coccygeal (with reference to vertebrae); drug coefficient
cd candela (SI)
CD$_{50}$ median curative dose (that which abolishes symptoms in 50% of test subjects
^{115}Cd radioactive cadmium
CDA chenodeoxycholic acid; completely denatured alcohol
CDAA chloro-diallylacetamide
CDAI Crohn's disease activity index
C&DB cough and deep-breathe
CDC calculated date of confinement; cell division cycle; Center for Disease Control (formerly Communicable Disease Center of HEW, Atlanta)
CD-C controlled drinker – control
CDCA chenodeoxycholic acid
CDD chronic disabling dermatosis
CDE canine distemper encephalitis
CD-E controlled drinker – experimental
CDP collagenase-digestible protein; Coronary Drug Project; cystosine diphosphate; cytidine diphosphate
CDPC cytidine diphosphate choline
CDPG Coronary Drug Project Group
CDS Chemical Data Systems

CDSM Committee on Dental and Surgical Materials (Brit)

CDT carbon dioxide therapy; Certified Dental Technician

Cdyn dynamic lung compliance (pulmonary function)

CE California encephalitis; cardiac enlargement; chemical energy; chick embryo; conjugated estrogens; constant error; Continuing Education; contractile element (of skeletal muscle); cytopathic effect

C/E Church of England

C-E chloroform-ether (mixture)

CEA carcinoembryonic antigen

CEC ciliated epithelial cells

CED Council on Education for the Deaf

CEENU CCNU

CeeNU CCNU

CEF centrifugation extractable fluid; chick embryo fibroblast

CEFMG Council on Education for Foreign Medical Graduates

CEI converting enzyme inhibitor

cej cement-enamel junction

Cel Celsius (thermometric scale)

cell celluloid (dentistry)

CELO chicken embryo lethal orphan (virus)

CEM conventional-transmission electron microscope

CEN Certification for Emergency Nursing

cen central

cent centigrade; central

CEO chick embryo origin

CEP Continuing Education Program; cortical evoked potential; countercurrent electrophoresis

CEPA chloroethane phosphoric acid

ceph-floc cephalin flocculation (test)

CEQ Council on Environmental Quality

CER ceramide; conditioned emotional response

CERD chronic end-stage renal disease

CERP Continuing Education Reeducation Program

cert certificate; certified

cerv cervical; cervix

CES central excitatory state

CESD cholesterol ester storage disease

CETI Communication with Extraterrestrial Intelligence

CF calibration factor; cancer-free; carbolfuchsin; carbon filtered; cardiac failure; Carworth Farms; chemotactic factor; chest and left leg lead; chick fibroblast; Christmas factor (PTC); citrovorum factor (folinic acid); colicin factor; colony forming; complement fixation; coronary flow; counting fingers; cycling fibroblast; cystic fibrosis

cf *confer* (L) compare with or refer to

c/f coloured female

CFA complement-fixing antibody; complete Freund's adjuvant

C-factor cleverness factor (psychology)

CFCCT Committee for Freedom of Choice in Cancer Therapy

CFD Concern for the Dying

CFF critical fusion or flicker frequency; Cystic Fibrosis Foundation

CFH Council on Family Health

CFI chemotactic factor inactivator; complement fixation inhibition (test)

CFM chlorofluoromethane (fluorocarbon)

cfm cubic feet per minute

CFMA Council for Medical Affairs

CFMG Commission on Foreign Medical Graduates

CFP cystic fibrosis of the pancreas

CFR case-fatality ratio; citrovorum-factor rescue

CFS Cystic Fibrosis Society

cfs cubic feet per second

CFSE crystal field stabilization energy

CFSTI Clearinghouse for Federal Scientific and Technical Information (later NTIS)

CFT complement-fixation test

CFU colony-forming unit

CFU-C colony-forming unit – culture

CFU-E colony-forming unit – erythroid

CFU-GM colony-forming unit – granulocyte macrophage

CFU-L colony-forming unit – lymphoid

CFU-M colony-forming unit – megakaryocyte

CFU-S colony-forming unit – haematopoietic (spleen)

CFW Carworth Farm mice (Webster strain)

CFX circumflex coronary artery

CG choking gas (phosgene); chorionic gonadotrophin; control group; cryoglobulin; cystine guanine; iodocyanine green

cg centigram (SI); centre of gravity

CGD chronic granulomatous disease; commissural gastric driver

CGFNS Commission on Graduates of Foreign Nursing Schools
CGH chorionic gonadotrophic hormone
CGI carbimazole
CGL chronic granulocytic leukaemia
CGM central grey matter (of spinal cord)
cgm centigram
CGN chronic glomerulonephritis
CGNB composite ganglioneuroblastoma
CGP N-carbobenzoxy-glycyl-L-phenylalanine; chorionic growth-hormone prolactin; circulating granulocyte pool
CGS catgut suture
CGS unit centimetre-gram-second unit
CH Certified Herbalist; *chirurgiae* (L) surgery; Christchurch chromosome; crown-heel (with reference to length of fetus)
C&H cocaine and heroin
Ch chapter; check; chest; Chido (antibodies); chief; child; choline
cH hydrogen ion concentration
CHA Catholic Hospital Association; chronic haemolytic anaemia; congenital hypoplastic anaemia; cyclohexyladenosine
ChA choline acetylase
CHAP Certified Hospital Admission Program
chap chapter
chart *charta* (L) a paper
chart bib *charta bibula* (L) blotting paper
chart cerat *charta cerata* (L) waxed paper
CHB complete heart block
ChB *Chirurgiae Baccalaureus* (L) Bachelor of Surgery
CHBA congenital Heinz body haemolytic anaemia
CHC Community Health Center; Community Health Computing; Community Health Council
CHCA Corresponding Health Care Associates
CHCP Correctional Health Care Program
CHD Chediak-Higashi disease; childhood disease; coronary heart disease
ChD *Chirurgiae Doctor* (L) Doctor of Surgery
ChE cholinesterase
CHEC Community Hypertension Evaluation Clinic
CHEF Chinese hamster embryo fibroblasts
chem chemistry(-ical)
CHF chick heart fibroblast; congestive heart failure

chg change
CHIP Comprehensive Health Insurance Plan
Chir Doct *Chirurgiae Doctor* (L) Doctor of Surgery
CHL chlorambucil
Chl chloroform
CHLA cyclohexyl linoleic acid
Chlb chlorobutanol
ChM *Chirurgiae Magister* (L) Master of Surgery
CHN carbon, hydrogen, nitrogen; Child Neurology
CHO carbohydrate
Cho choline
chol cholesterol
chol est cholesterol esters
CHP Child Psychiatry; Comprehensive Health Planning
  (HHS)
ChP Chest Physician
chpx chickenpox
CHR cercarienhullenreaktion
Chr *Chromobacterium*
chr chronic
c hr candle hour
ChrBrSyn chronic brain syndrome
Chron chronical
CHSD Children's Health Services Division (HHS)
CHSS Cooperative Health Statistics System
ChTg chymotrypsinogen
ChTK chicken thymidine kinase
CI cardiac index; cephalic index; chemotherapeutic in-
  dex; clonus index; coefficient of intelligence; colour in-
  dex; contamination index; coronary insufficiency; cor-
  rected count increment; crystalline insulin; cytotoxic
  index
Ci curie
CIA chymotrypsin inhibitor activity
cib *cibus* (L) food
CIBHA congenital inclusion body haemolytic anaemia
CIC cardiac inhibitory centre; circulating immune com-
  plexes
CICU Cardiovascular In-patient Care Unit; Coronary In-
  tensive Care Unit
CID chick infective dose; cytomegalic inclusion disease
CIE countercurrent immunoelectrophoresis
CIEP counterimmuno-electrophoresis
CIF cloning inhibiting factor
CIFC Council for the Investigation of Fertility Control

cIgM cytoplasmic immunoglobulin M
CIH carbohydrate-induced hyperglyceridaemia; Certificate in Industrial Health; Children in Hospitals
CIM cortically induced movement; Cumulated Index Medicus
CIN cervical intraepithelial neoplasia
CIOMS Council for International Organizations of Medical Sciences
cir circular
circ circuit; circular; circulatory; circumcision(ed)
CIRM Centro Internazionale Radio-Medico
CIS central inhibitory state; Chemical Information System
cit citrate
cito disp *cito dispensetur* (L) dispense quickly
CJD Creutzfeldt-Jakob disease
CK choline kinase; creatine kinase; cyanogen chloride; cytokinin
ck check(ed)
CL cardiolipin; chest and left arm lead (cardiology); chronic leukaemia; cholesterol-lecithin (test); Clinical Laboratory; corpus luteum; critical list
CLA cervicolinguoaxial
Cl chloride; chlorine; clavicle; clinic; *Clostridium;* closure; colistin
cl centilitre (SI)
CLA cyclic lysine anhydride
ClAc chloroacetyl
class classification
CLB chlorambucil
cldy cloudy
CLED cystine-lactose electrolyte deficient
Clin clinical
clini clinitest
Clin path clinical pathology
Clin proc clinical procedures
CLIP corticotrophin-like intermediate lobe peptide
CLL cholesterol-lowering lipid; chronic lymphocytic leukaemia
Cl liq clear liquid
CLO cod liver oil
ClO chlorine monoxide
Clon *Clonorchis*
ClP Clinical Pathology
cl pal cleft palate

CLR chloride test (dentistry)

CLT chronic lymphocytic thyroiditis; clot lysis time

CM California mastitis (test); carboxymethyl; cardiomyopathy; Chick-Martin (coefficient); *Chirurgiae Magister* (L) Master in Surgery; chopped meat (medium); circular muscle; cochlear microphonics; complete medium (microbiology); congenital malformation; congestive myocardiopathy; contrast medium; copulatory mechanism

C&M cocaine and morphine mixed

C_m maximum clearance (with reference to urea clearance test)

cm centimetre (SI); costal margin; *cras mane* (L) tomorrow morning

cm^3 cubic centimetre (SI)

CMA Canadian Medical Association

CMB carbolic methylene blue; Central Midwives' Board; chloromercuribenzoate

CMC carboxymethyl cellulose; carpometacarpal; cell-mediated cytolysis

CMD childhood muscular dystrophy; count median diameter (of particles)

CME crude marijuana extract; continuing medical education

CMF Christian Medical Fellowship (Brit); chondromyxoid fibroma; cortical magnification factor; cyclophosphamide, methotrexate, 5-fluorouracil

CMG chopped meat glucose (agar); cystometrography

CMH congenital malformation of heart

CMHC Community Mental Health Center

CMI carbohydrate metabolism index; cell-mediated immunity; chronic mesenteric ischaemia; Commonwealth Mycological Institute; Cornell Medical Index

CMIT Current Medical Information and Technology

CMJ Committee on Medical Journalism

CMK chloromethyl ketone

CML cell-mediated lympholysis; chronic myelocytic leukaemia

cmm cubic millimetre

CMN cystic medial necrosis (of aorta)

CMO cardiac minute output; Chief Medical Officer (Brit); corticosterone methyl oxidase

CMP Competitive Medical Plans; Comprehensive Medical Plan; cytidine monophosphate

CMR cerebral metabolic rate

CMRG cerebral metabolic rate for glucose

CMRO₂ cerebral metabolic rate for oxygen

CMS Christian Medical Society

cms *cras mane sumendus* (L) to be taken tomorrow morning

cm/s centimetre per second

CMSS circulation, motor ability, sensation and swelling

CMT California mastitis test; Council on Medical Television; Current Medical Terminology

CMV cytomegalovirus

CN caudate nucleus; cellulose nitrate; Charge Nurse; child nutrition; chloroacetophenone; clinical nursing; cochlear nucleus (of the brain); cranial nerve; cyanogen radical

C/N carbon to nitrogen ratio

cn *cras nocte* (L) tomorrow night

CNA Canadian Nurses' Association

CNB cutting needle biopsy

CNCBL cyanocobalamin

CNE chronic nervous exhaustion

CNM Certified Nurse-Midwife

CNR Civil Nursing Reserve; Council of National Representatives (of International Council of Nurses)

CNS central nervous system; sulphocyanate

cns *cras nocte sumendus* (L) to be taken tomorrow night

CNSHA congenital nonspherocytic haemolytic anaemia

CNV colistimethate, nystatin, vancomycin

CO carbon monoxide; cardiac output; castor oil; casualty officer; centric occlusion; choline oxidase; crossover(s) (genetics)

C/O check out; complains of

CO₂ carbon dioxide

Co cobalt; coenzyme

⁶⁰Co radioactive cobalt

co *compositus* (L) a compound, compounded

CO I coenzmne I, diphosphopyridine nucleotide (DPN)

CO II coenzyme II, triphosphopyridine nucleotide (TPN)

CoA coenzyme A

COAD chronic obstructive airway disease

coag coagulate(-ation)

COBT chronic obstruction of biliary tract

COC cathodal opening contraction; coccygeal; combination (type) oral contraceptive

coch, cochleat *cochlear, cochleare, cochleatum* (L) a

spoonful, by spoonfuls

coch amp *cochleare amplum* (L) tablespoon

coch mag *cochleare magnum* (L) a large spoonful (about 14 ml)

coch med *cochleare medium* (L) a dessert spoonful (about 7 ml)

coch parv *cochleare parvum* (L) a teaspoonful (about 4 ml)

COCI Consortium on Chemical Information (Brit)

COCl cathodal opening clonus

coct *coctio* (L) boiling

COD cause of death; chemical oxygen demand; Council of Deans

cod codeine

coeff coefficient

COEPS cortically originating extrapyramidal system

CoF cobra factor

COGTT cortisone (primed) oral glucose tolerance test

COH carbohydrate

COHb carboxyhaemoglobin

col *cola* (L) strain; colony (bacteriology); coloured; column

colat *colatus* (L) strained

COLD chronic obstructive lung disease

colen *colentur* (L) let them be strained

colet *coleatur* (L) let it be strained

coll collect(ion); college; colloidal; *collyrium* (L) an eyewash

collun *collunarium* (L) nose wash

collut *collutorium* (L) a mouthwash

coll vol collective volume

collyr *collyrium* (L) an eyewash

COM College of Osteopathic Medicine

commun dis communicable disease

comp compare; compensated; complaint; composition; *compositus* (L) compounded of; compound

Comp case Compensation (*workman's*) case

compd compound

compl completed; complications

Complic complications

compn composition

COMT catecholamine-O-methyltransferase

COMTRAC computer-based case tracing

con *contra* (L) against

conc concentration(-ated)

cond concentrated
concentr concentrated
concis *concisus* (L) cut
cocn concentration(-trate)
cond condensed; condition(s); conductivity
cond ref conditioned reflex
cond resp conditioned response
conf *confectio* (L) a confection; conference
cong *congius* (L) gallon
congen congenital
conj conjunctiva
Cons consultant, consulting
cons *conserva* (L) keep, save; *consonans* (L) tinkling
consperg *consperge* (L) dust, sprinkle
const constant
constit constituent; constitution(-al)
cont containing; contents; continue; *contra* (L) against; *contusus* (L) bruised
contag contagious
conter *contere* (L) rub together
contg containing
contin *continuetur* (L) let it be continued
contra contraindicated
contralat contralateral
cont rem *continuantur remedia* (L) let the medicine be continued
contrit *contritus* (L) broken, ground
contus *contusus* (L) bruised
conv convalescent
conv strab convergent strabismus
COOD chronic obstructive outflow disease
COOH carboxyl group
coord coordination
COP change of plaster; colloidal osmotic pressure; cyclophosphamide, oncovin (vincristine) and prednisone
COPC Community Oriented Primary Care
COPD chronic obstructive pulmonary disease
COPE chronic obstructive pulmonary emphysema
COPRO coproporphyrin
COQ ubiquinone (coenzyme Q)
coq *coque* (L) to boil
coq in sa *coque in sufficiente aqua* (L) boil in sufficient water
coq sa *coque secundum artem* (L) boil properly

coq simul (L) boil together

COR cardiac output recorder; *corpus* (L) body; corrosive; cortisone

CoR Congo red

cor corrected(-tion)

CORD Commissioned Officer Residency Deferment (Program)

cort cortex, cortical

COS Canadian Ophthalmological Society; Clinical Orthopedic Society

COSPAR Committee on Space Research

COSTEP Commissioned Officer Student Training and Extern Program

COT colony overlay test; contralateral optic tectum

COTA Certified Occupational Therapy Assistant

COTe cathodal opening tetanus

COV cross-over value (genetics)

CoVF cobra venom factor

COWS cold to the opposite and warm to the same side (audiometry)

CP candle power; capillary pressure; cerebral palsy; Certified Prosthetist; chemically pure; Child Psychiatry; Child Psychology; choloroquine-primaquine; chronic pyelonephritis; cleft palate; Clinical Pathology; cochlear potential; code of practice; colour perception; combining power; compensated base; compound; compressed (tablet); constant pressure; coproporphyrin; corocoid process; cor pulmonale (right ventricular failure); creatine phosphate (phosphocreatine); crude protein; current practice

C/P cholesterol-phospholipid ratio

C&P compensation and pension; cystoscopy and pyelogram

Cp chickenpox

cp centipoise; compare

CPA Canadian Psychiatric Association; chlorophenylalanine; circulating platelet aggregate

CPAF chlorpropamide-alcohol flushing

CPAH *p*-aminohippuric acid clearance

CPAP continuous positive airway pressure

CPB cardiopulmonary bypass; cetyl pyridinium bromide; competitive protein-binding

CPBA competitive protein-binding analysis

CPC Cerebral Palsy Clinic; chronic passive congestion; Clinical Pathological Conference; circumferential pneumatic compression

CPCL congenital pulmonary cystic lymphangiectasis

CPCP chronic progressive coccidioidal pneumonitis

CPD cephalopelvic disproportion; citrate phosphate dextrose; contact potential difference; contagious pustular dermatitis; cyclopentadiene

CPDD cis-platinum-diamine-dichloride

CPE chronic pulmonary emphysema; corona penetrating enzyme; cytopathogenic effects

CPH Certificate in Public Health

CPH 5 Cutter protein hydrolysate, 5% in water

CPHA Commission on Professional and Hospital Activities

CPHE crew personal hygiene equipment

CPI Cancer Potential Index (Environmental Monitoring); California Psychological Inventory; constitutional psychopathia inferior

CPIB chlorophenoxyisobutyrate

CPK creatine phosphokinase

cpl complete

CPLM cysteine-peptone-liver infusion (media)

CPM central pontine myelinolysis; chlorpheniramine maleate; counts per minute

CPP carboxy terminus of propressophysin; cerebral perfusion pressure; cyclopenteno-phenanthrene

CPPB constant positive pressure breathing

CPPD calcium pyrophosphate dihydrate

CPPV continuous positive pressure ventilation

CPR cardiac pulmonary reserve; cardiopulmonary resuscitation; centripetal rub; chlorophenyl red

CPRD Committee on Prosthetics Research and Development

CPS C-polysaccharide; constitutional psychopathic state

cps cycles (double vibrations) per second

CPT ciliary particle transport activity; combining power test; continuous performance test; Current Procedural Terminology

CPU central processing unit

CPUE chest pain of unknown etiology

CPZ chlorpromazine

CQ chloroquine; conceptual quotient

CQM chloroquine mustard

CR cardiorespiratory; centric relation; cephalothin; chest and right arm (lead); chest roentgenogram; Clinical Record; clot retraction; coefficient of fat retention;

colon resection; complement receptor; complete remission; complete response; conditioned reflex or response; cresyl red; critical ratio; crown-rump (with reference to length of fetus)

C&R Convalescent and Rehabilitation

Cr chromium; cranial; creatinine; crown

^{51}Cr radioactive sodium chromate

cr *cras* (L) tomorrow

Cr&Br crown and bridge

CRA central retinal artery; Chinese restaurant asthma

CRABP cellular retinoic acid-binding protein

CRAO central retinal artery occlusion

crast *crastinus* (L) for tomorrow

CRB chemical, radiological, and biological (warfare)

CRBBB complete right bundle branch block

CRC calomel, rhubarb, colocynth; cardiovascular reflex conditioning; Clinical Research Centre (MRC)

CRCS cardiovascular reflex conditioning system

CRD chronic renal disease; chronic respiratory disease; complete reaction of degeneration

CRE cumulative radiation effect

crep *crepitus* (L) crepitation

CREST calcinosis, Raynaud's phenomenon, esophageal dysfunction, sclerodactyly, and telangiectasia

CRF chronic renal failure; coagulase reacting factor; corticotrophin(ACTH)-releasing factor

CRH corticotrophin(ACTH)-releasing hormone

CRHL Collaborative Radiological Health Laboratory

CRI chemical rust inhibiting (germicide); cold running intelligibility (with reference to test for hearing continuous speech); cross-reactive idiotype (genetics)

CRL Certified Record Librarian; complement receptor lymphocyte; crown-rump length

CRM Certified Reference Materials; cross-reacting material

Cr nn cranial nerves

CRO cathode ray oscilloscope; centric relation occlusion

CROS contralateral routing of signal

CRP C-reactive protein

CrP creatine phosphate

CRPA C-reactive protein antiserum

CRS Chinese restaurant syndrome; colon and rectal surgery; congenital rubella syndrome

CRST calcinosis, Raynaud's Phenomenon, sclerodactyly, telangiectasis

CRT cardiac resuscitation team; cathode ray tube; complex reaction timer

CRTP Consciousness Research and Training Project

CRTT Certified Respiratory Therapy Technician

CRU Clinical Research Unit

CRVS California Relative Value Studies

crys crystalline(-ized)

cryst crystalline(-ized)

CS Caesarean section; Central Supply; cerebrospinal; cervical stimulation; chest strap; chondroitin sulphate; chorionic somatomammotrophin; Christian Scientist; Church of Scotland; clinical state; *colla sinistra* (L) with the left hand; concentrated strength (of solutions); conditioned stimulus; congenital syphilis; conscious(ness); convalescent status; coronary sclerosis; corticosteroid; current strength; cycloserine

C&S culture and sensitivity

Cs caesium; case(s); Cost-Stirling antibodies; standard clearance (with reference to urea clearance test)

¹³⁷Cs radioactive caesium

cS centistoke

CSA chondroitin sulphate A; colony-stimulating activity; cyclosporin A

CSC collagen sponge contraceptive; cryogenic storage container

csc *coup sur coup* (L) in small doses at short intervals

CSCD Center for Sickle Cell Disease

CSCR Central Society for Clinical Research

CSD cat-scratch disease; conditionally streptomycin dependent; cortically spreading depression; Doctor of Christian Science

CSF cerebrospinal fluid; colony stimulating factor

CSFR Committee on Scientific Freedom and Responsibility

CSF-WR cerebrospinal fluid – Wassermann reaction

CSI cancer serum index

CSICU Cardiac Surgical Intensive Care Unit

CSM cerebrospinal meningitis; Committee on Safety of Medicines

CSMB Center for the Study of Multiple Births

CSMMG Chartered Society of Massage and Medical Gymnastics

CSOM chronic suppurative otitis media

CSP Chartered Society of Physiotherapy; Cooperative Statistical Program (for IUD data); criminal sexual psychopath

CSPI Center for Science in the Public Interest

CSR Cheyne-Stokes respiration; corrected sedimentation rate; cortical secretion rate (of adrenal)

CSS chewing, sucking, swallowing; chronic subclinical scurvy

CSSD Central Sterile Supply Department

CST cavernous sinus thrombosis; contraction stress test (gynaecology); convulsive shock therapy

Cstat static lung compliance

CSTI Clearinghouse for Scientific and Technical Information

CStJ Commander, Order of St John of Jerusalem

CSU catheter specimen of urine; Central Statistical Unit (of VDRL)

CT calcitonin; carpal tunnel; Cellular Therapy; cerebral thrombosis; cholera toxin; chymotrypsin; clotting (coagulation) time; coated tablet; compressed tablet; computerized tomography; connective tissue; continue treatment; continuous-flow tub; contraceptive techniques; controlled temperature; corneal transplant; coronary thrombosis; corrective therapist(-apy); cystine-tellurite (medium); cytotechnologist

Ct *Ctenocephalides*

CTA Canadian Tuberculosis Association; cyano-trimethyl-androsterone; cyproterone acetate; cystine trypticase agar

CTa catamenia (menstruation)

CTAB cetyltrimethyl-ammonium bromide

CTAC Cancer Treatment Advisory Committee (HHS)

ctant *cum tanto* (L) with the same amount of

CTAP connective tissues activating peptides

CTC chlortetracycline; Clinical Trial Certificate (Brit)

CTCL cutaneous T-cell lymphoma

CTD carpal tunnel decompression; Convalescent Training Depot

CTEM conventional transmission electron microscope

CTF Cancer Therapy Facility; certificate; cytotoxic factor

CTG cardiotocography

CTL cytologic thymus-dependent lymphocyte

CTM cardiotachometer

CTMM computed tomographic metrizamide myelography

CTP cytidine triphosphate; cytosine triphosphate

CTR cardiothoracic ratio

ctr centre

CTS carpal tunnel syndrome; computerized topographic scanner

CTT compressed tablet triturate; computerized trans-axial tomogram

CTU Cardiac/Thoracic Unit; centigrade thermal unit

CTX cefotaxime; cerebrotendinous xanthomatosis

CTZ chemoreceptor trigger zone (vomiting area in medulla)

CU clinical unit; chymotrypsin unit; Convalescent Unit

Cu copper

^{61}Cu, ^{64}Cu radioactive copper

cu cubic

CuB copper band (dentistry)

CUC chronic ulcerative colitis

cu cm cubic centimetre

CUG cystidine-uridine-guanidine; cystourethrogram

cuj *cujus* (L) of which, of any

cuj lib *cujus libet* (L) of whatever you please

cult culture (bacteriology)

CUMITECH Cumulative Techniques and Procedures in Clinical Microbiology

cu mm cubic millimetre

cu mu cubic micrometre

CUP Care Unit Program (against alcoholism)

cur curative; current

curat *curatio* (L) a dressing

CURN Conduct and Utilization of Research in Nursing

CuSCN cuprous thiocyanate

CV cardiovascular; cell volume; cerebrovascular; cervical vertebra; closing volume; coefficient of variation; colour vision; concentrated volume (solutions); *conjugata vera* (L) true conjugate diameter of pelvic inlet; conversational voice; corpuscular volume; *cras vespere* (L) tomorrow evening; cresyl violet; crystal violet

Cv specific heat at constant volume

CVA cerebrovascular accident

cva costovertebral angle

CVC Convalescent Camp

CVD cardiovascular disease; colour vision deviate

CVDS Cardiomuscular Disease Study (Brit)

CVF central visual field

CVI common variable immunodeficiency

CVM cardiovascular monitor

CVMP Committee on Veterans Medical Problems
CVO Chief Veterinary Officer; *conjugata vera obstetrica* (L) obstetric conjugate diameter
CVP cell volume profile; central venous pressure; cyclophosphamide, vincristine and prednisone
CVR cardiovascular renal (disease); cardiovascular-respiratory; cephalic vasomotor response; cerebrovascular resistance
CVS cardiovascular surgery; cardiovascular system; clean voided specimen
CVTR charcoal viral transport medium
CW case work; cell wall; chemical warfare; chest wall; Children's Ward; clockwise; continuous wave; crutch walking
CWBTS capillary whole blood true sugar
CWD cell wall defective
CWI cardiac work index
CWOP childbirth without pain
CWP coal worker's pneumoconiosis
CWPEA Childbirth Without Pain Education Association
CWS Child Welfare Service; cold-water soluble
CWT cold water treatment
cwt hundredweight
CX cervix; chest X-ray
Cx clearance (physiology); convex
CXR Chest X-ray
Cy cyanogen
CYA Cyclosporin A
cyath *cyathus* (L) a glass
cyath vin *cyathus vinarius* (L) a wineglass
CYC cyclophosphamide
cyc cyclazocine; cycle; cyclotron
CYE charcoal yeast extract (medium)
CYL casein yeast lactate (media)
cyl cylinder; cylindrical lens
CYN cyanide
CYS cystoscopy
Cys cysteine
Cys-cys cystine
cytol cytology(-ological)
cyt sys cytochrome system
CZ cefazolin
CZI crystalline zinc insulin

D

D   symbol for vitamin D potency of good cod-liver oil; *da* (L) give; date; daughter; dead, deceased; dead air space; deciduous; degree; dental; *dentur* (L) let such be given; dermatologist(-ology); *detur* (L) let it be given; deuterium (heavy hydrogen); developed (*see* w/d); deviation; diagnosis; diameter; died; difference; diffuse; diffusing capacity; diffusion constant; dioptre; disease; divorced; dog (veterinary medicine); donor; Doriden (glutethimide); dorsal; *dosis* (L) dose; drive or drive state; drug; duodenum; dwarf

d   dead; deci (prefix) (SI); density; dexter (right); dextrorotatory; died, deceased; *dies* (L) day; dioptre; distal; dorsal; dose; doubtful; duration

δ,Δ   delta

D-   dextrorotatory; A chemical prefix (small capital) which designates that a substance has the configuration of D-glyceraldehyde; In carbohydrate nomenclature, the symbol designates the configuration family of the *highest numbered* asymmetric carbon atom, as in D-glucose; In amino acid nomenclature, the symbol designates the configuration family of the *lowest numbered* asymmetric carbon atom, as in D-threonine

d-   Chemical abbreviation for *dextro*, to the right or clockwise, especially with reference to direction in which a plane of polarized light is rotated

D_1, D_2, etc   first dorsal (thoracic) vertebra, second dorsal vertebra, etc

17-D   a modified yellow fever virus

D 860   tolbutamide

D_0   diffusing capacity of oxygen

DA   degenerative arthritis; delayed action (with reference to drugs); Dental Assistant; developmental age; diphenylchlorarsine; Diploma in Anaesthetics; disability assistance; District Administrator; dopaminergic; drug addict

D/A   discharge and advise

D-A   donor-acceptor

da   daughter; day; deca (prefix) (SI)

DAB   dysrhythmic aggressive behaviour

DAC   Disaster Assistance Center; Disablement Advisory Committee (Brit); Division of Ambulatory Care

DACT   dactinomycin (actinomycin D)

DAD   dispense as directed

DADAVS Deputy Assistant Director Army Veterinary Services

DADDS diacetyl diaminodiphenylsulphone (acedapsone)

DADLE D-Ala, D-Leu enkephalin

DADPS diphenylsulphone (dapsone)

DADMS Deputy Assistant Director of Medical Services (Armed Forces)

DADS Director Army Dental Service

DAE diphenylanthracene endoperoxide

DAF delayed auditory feedback

DAH disordered action of the heart

DAHEA Department of Allied Health Education and Accreditation (AMA)

DAHM Division of Allied Health Manpower

DALA delta-aminolaevulinic acid

DALE Drug Abuse Law Enforcement

DAM degraded amyloid; diacetyl monoxime; diacetyl-morphine; Dictionary of Abbreviations in Medicine

dam decametre (SI)

dAMP deoxyadenylate adenosine monophosphate

dand *dandus* (L) to be given

DAO duly authorized officer

DAP diaminopimelic acid; dihydroxyacetone phosphate; direct latex agglutination pregnancy (test); Director of Army Psychiatry (Brit); draw a person test

DAP&E Diploma of Applied Parasitology and Entomology

DAPRU Drug Abuse Prevention Resource Unit

DARTS Drug and Alcohol Rehabilitation Testing System

DAS dextroamphetamine sulphate

DASH Distress Alarm for the Severely Handicapped (Brit)

DAT delayed action tablet; Dental Admission Test; diet as tolerated; differential agglutination titre; differential aptitude test; Disaster Action Team (Red Cross)

dau daughter

DAV Disabled American Veterans

DAV&RS Director Army Veterinary and Remount Services

DAvMed Diploma in Aviation Medicine

DAyM Doctor of Ayurvedic Medicine

DB Baudelocque's diameter (external conjugate diameter of pelvis); diet beverage; distobuccal; dry bulb; Dutch belted (rabbits)

dB decibel (SI)

db decibel
DBA dibenzanthracene
DBC dye-binding capacity
DBD dibromodulcitol (mitolactol)
DBE dibromoethane (ethylene dibromide)
DBI development at birth index; phenformin
DBK decarboxylase base Moeller; diabetic management; dibromomannitol (mitobronitol)
DBO distobucco-occlusal
DBP diastolic blood pressure; dibutylphthalate; distobuccopulpal
DBS despeciated bovine serum; Division of Biological Standards
DBT dry bulb temperature
DBW desirable body weight
DC Dental Corps; diagnostic centre; digit copying; diphenylcyanoarsine; direct current; discharged; discontinue; distocervical; Doctor of Chiropractic; donor's cells (corpuscles)
D/C discontinue
D&C dilatation and curettage; Drugs and Cosmetics
DCA deoxycholic acid; desoxycholate citrate agar; deoxycorticosterone acetate; dichloroacetate
DCC Day Care Center; Disaster Control Center
DCc double concave
DC$_{co}$ diffusing capacity for carbon dioxide
DCD Diploma in Chest Diseases (Brit)
DCF deoxycoformycin; direct centrifugal flotation
DCG deoxycorticosterone glucoside
DCH Diploma in Child Health
DCh *Doctor Chirurgiae* (L) Doctor of Surgery
DCHN dicyclohexylamine nitrite
DChO Doctor of Ophthalmic Surgery (Brit)
DCI dichloroisoprenaline; dichloroisoproterenol
DCLS deoxycholate citrate lactose saccharose (agar)
DCM dichloromethane; Doctor of Comparative Medicine
DCMT Doctor of Clinical Medicine of the Tropics (Brit)
DCN delayed conditioned necrosis; dorsal cutaneous nerve
DCNU chlorozotocin
DCO Diploma of the College of Optics (Brit)
DCP dicalcium phosphate; Diploma in Clinical Pathology; Diploma in Clinical Psychology; District Community Physician

DCR dacryocystorhinostomy; direct cortical response

DCS dense canalicular system; Doctor of Christian Science; dorsal column stimulator

DCT diastolic control team; direct Coombs's test; distal convoluted tubule (of kidney)

DCTMA deoxycorticosterone-trimethyl-acetate

DCU dichloral urea

DCVO Deputy Chief Veterinary Officer

DCx double convex

DD dangerous drug; *de die* (L) daily; degenerative disease; dependent drainage; developmental disability; differential diagnosis; disc diameter; discharged dead; double diffusion (test); dry dressing

DDA An acetic derivative of DDT excreted in urine; Dangerous Drugs Act; dideoxyadenosine

DDAVP deamino-D-arginine vasopressin

DDC dangerous drug cabinet; diethyldithiocarbamate

DDD dehydroxydinaphthyl disulphide; dichlorodiphenyl-dichloro-ethane

DDG deoxy-D-glucose

DDH Diploma in Dental Health (Brit)

DDIB Disease Detection Information Bureau

dd in d *de die in diem* (L) from day to day

DDM Diploma in Dermatological Medicine; Doctor of Dental Medicine

DDMS Deputy Director of Medical Services (Armed Forces)

DDO Diploma in Dental Orthopaedics

DDR Diploma in Diagnostic Radiology

DDRB Doctors' and Dentists' Review Body (Brit)

DDS dialysis disequilibrium syndrome; diamino-diphenyl-sulphone (dapsone); Director of Dental Services; Doctor of Dental Science; Doctor of Dental Surgery

DDSc Doctor of Dental Science

DDSO diamino-diphenyl-sulphoxide

DDST Denver Developmental Screening Test

DDT dichloro-diphenyl-trichloro-ethane; ductus deferens tumour

DE deprived eye (optics); digestive energy; drug evaluation

D&E dilatation and evacuation

DEA dehydroepiandrosterone; Drug Enforcement Administration

DEAE diethylaminoethanol

dearg pil *deargentur pilulae* (L) let the pills be silverized
deaur pil *deaurentur pilulae* (L) let the pills be gilded
DEB diethylbutanediol; Division of Environmental Biology
DEBRA Dystrophic Epidermolysis Bullosa Research Association
deb spis *debita spissitudine* (L) of the proper consistency
DEC diethylcarbamazine; dynamic environmental conditioning (cycle)
dec *decanta* (L) pour off; decompose; decrease
decd deceased; dead
decoct *decoctum* (L) decoction
decomp decompose, decomposition
dec (R) decrease, relative
decr decreased or diminished
decub *decubitus* (L) lying down
DED date of expected delivery; delayed erythema dose
de d in d *de die in diem* (L) from day to day
DEF Dental formula designating: number of teeth for filling; e, number for extraction; f, number of filled teeth (with reference to deciduous teeth)
def defecation; deficient; define(-inition)
defib defibrillate
defic deficiency; deficit
deform deformity
deg degeneration; degree
degen degeneration
deglut *deglutiatur* (L) let it be swallowed
DEHS Division of Emergency Health Services
dej dentoenamel junction
Del delivery
del delusion
deliq deliquescent
Dem Demerol (pethidine hydrochloride)
denat denatured
Dent dental; dentistry; dentition
dent *dentur* (L) give, let it be given
dent tal dos *dentur tales doses* (L) give of such doses
DEP diethylpropanediol
Dep dependants
dep *deputatus* (L) purified
DEPA diethylene phosphoramide
depr depressed
DeR reaction of degeneration
deriv derivative of, derived from

Derm dermatology(-ologist, -itis)

DES diethylstilboestrol; diffuse esophageal spasm; Doctor's Emergency Service

desat desaturated

desc descendent(-ding)

dest *destilla* (L) distil and *distillatus* (L) distilled

destil *destilla* (L) distil

DET diethyltryptamine

det *detur* (L) let it be given

determin determination

det in dup *detur in duplo* (L) let twice as much be given

det in 2 plo *detur in duplo* (L) let twice as much be given

detn detention

d et s *detur et signatur* (L) let it be given and labelled

DEV duck egg (embryo) virus or vaccine

dev deviation

devel develop(ment)

DF decapacitation factor (with reference to sperm); decontamination factor; deferoxamine mesylate; degree of freedom (of movement); Dermatology Foundation; dietary fibre; dorsiflexion

DFB dinitrofluorobenzene; dysfunctional uterine bleeding

DFC dry-filled capsules

DFDT difluoro-diphenyl-trichloro-ethane

DFHom Diploma of the Faculty of Homoeopathy

DFI disease-free intervals

DFL Doctor of Family Life

DFMO difluoromethyl ornithine

DFMR daily fetal movements record

DFO District Finance Officer

DFP diastolic filling period; diisopropyl fluorophosphate (dyflos)

DFSP dermatofibrosarcoma protuberans

DG deoxy-D-glucose; diagnosis; diglyceride; distogingival

dG deoxyguanylate

dg decigram (SI)

DGMS Director General of Medical Services (Armed Forces); Division of General Medical Sciences

DGO Diploma in Gynaecology & Obstetrics

DGR Director of Graves Registration (Brit)

DGV dextrose-gelatin-veronal solution

DH Day Hospital; dehydrogenase; delayed hypersensitivity; dermatitis herpetiformis; disseminated histoplasmosis; dominant hand

D/H   deuterium to hydrogen ratio
DHA   dehydroepiandrosterone; dihydroacetic acid
DHAD   1, 4-dihydroxy-5, 8-bis [2-(2-hydroxyethyl-amino)ethylamino] anthraquinone dihydrochloride (mitoxantrone hydrochloride)
DHAS   dehydroepiandrosterone sulphate
DHBV   duck hepatic B virus
DHC   dehydrocholesterol; dehydrocholic acid
DHE   dihydroergotamine
DHEA   dihydroepiandrosterone
DHES   Division of Health Examination Statistics
DHEW   Department of Health, Education and Welfare (US), *now* DHHS
DHg   Doctor of Hygiene
DHHS   Department of Health and Human Science
DHI   Dental Health International; dihydroxyindol
DHIA   dehydroisoandrosterol
DHIC   dihydroisocodeine
DHK   dihydroergocryptine
DHM   dihydromorphine
DHMA   dehydroxymandelic acid
DHMSA   Diploma in History of Medicine, Society of Apothecaries
DHO   deuterium hydrogen (protium) oxide
DHO 180   dihydroergocornine
DHP   dehydrogenated polymers
DHPG   dehydroxyphenylglycol
dhPRL   decidual prolactin
DHR   delayed hypersensitivity reactions
D-5-HS   dextrose (5%) in Hartman's solution
DHSM   dihydrostreptomycin
DHSS   Department of Health and Social Security (UK); dihydrostreptomycin sulphate
DHT   dihydrotachysterol; dihydrotestosterone; dihydro-thymine
DHTB   dihydroteleocidin B
DHTP   dihydrotestosterone propionate
DHyg   Doctor of Hygiene
DHZ   dihydralazine
DI   defective-interfering; deterioration index; diabetes insipidus; distoincisal; double indemnity; drug information; drug interactions; dyskaryosis index
DIA   Drug Information Association
dia   diathermy
diab   diabetic

DIAC di-iodothyroacetic acid

diag diagnosis, diagnostic; diagonal; diagram

diam diameter

dias diastolic

diath diathermy

DIB butyl di-iodo-hydroxybenzoate

DIC differential interference contrast (microscope); 5-(3,3,dimethyl-1-triazeno)imidazole-4-carboxamide (dacarbazine); disseminated intravascular coagulopathy or coagulation

dick ethyldichloroarsine

dict dictionary

DIE direct injection enthalpimetry

dieb alt *diebus alternus* (L) on alternate days

dieb tert *diebus tertius* (L) every third day

diff difference; differential blood count

diff diag differential diagnosis

DIFP diisopropyl fluorophosphonate

Dig *digeratur* (L) let it be digested

DIH Diploma in Industrial Health

DIHPPA di-iodohydroxy-phenylpyruvic acid

dil *dilue, dilutus* (L) dilute, diluted

dilat dilatation, dilated

dild diluted

diln dilution

diluc *diluculo* (L) at daybreak

dilut *dilutus* (L) dilute

dim *dimidius* (L) one-half; *diminutus* (L) diminished

d in p aeq *divide in partes aequales* (L) divide into equal parts

DIP desquamative interstitial pneumonia; distal interphalangeal (joint)

Dip diploma, diplomate

DIPA di-isopropylamine

DipAmerBdP&N Diplomate American Board of Psychiatry and Neurology

DipBact Diploma in Bacteriology

DipChem Diploma in Chemistry (Brit)

DipClinPath Diploma in Clinical Pathology (Brit)

diph diphtheria

diph-tet diphtheria-tetanus

diph-tox diphtheria toxoid (plain)

diph-tox AP diphtheria toxoid (alum precipitated)

DipMicrobiol Diploma in Microbiology

DipSocMed Diploma in Social Medicine (Brit)

Dir   director
dir   *directione* (L) directions
dir prop   *directione propria* (L) with the proper directions
dis   disability, disabled; disease; distance
disc   discontinue
disch   discharge(d)
disloc   dislocation
disod   disodium
disp   *dispensa* (L) dispense; dispensary
diss   dissolve(d)
dissem   disseminated
dist   distance; *distilla* (L) distil
dist f   distinguished from
distn   distillation
DIT   diiodotyrosine
div   divergence; *divide* (L) divide; division; divorced
div in par aeq   *dividatur in partes aequales* (L) divide into equal parts
DJD   degenerative joint disease
dkg   dekagram
dkm   dekameter
DKTC   dog kidney tissue culture
DKV   deer kidney virus
DL   danger list; difference limen (threshold); disabled list; distolingual; Donath-Landsteiner (test)
dl   decilitre (SI)
DLa   distolabial
DLal   distolabioincisal
DLaP   distolabiopulpal
DLC   differential leucocyte count
DLCO₂   diffusing capacity for lung carbon dioxide
DLE   discoid lupus erythematosus
DLF   Disabled Living Foundation; dorsolateral funiculus
DLI   distolinguoincisal
DLLI   dulcitol lysine lactose iron (agar)
DLO   Diploma in Laryngology and Otology; distolinguo-occlusal
DLP   distolinguopulpal
DLT   dihydroepiandrosterone loading test
DLVO   Derjaguin-Landau-Verwey-Overbeek   theory (microbiology)
DM   dextromethorphan; diabetes mellitus; diastolic murmur; diphenylaminearsine chloride (Adamsite); *Doctor Medicinae* (L) Doctor of Medicine
dm   decimetre (SI)

DMA dimethylamine; dimethylarginine
DMAC dimethylacetamide
DMBA dimethylbenzanthracene
DMC demeclocycline; dimethylcarbinol; dimite (1, 1-bis-[*p*-chloro-phenyl] ethanol); direct microscopic count
DMCC direct microscopic clump count
DMCM dimethoxyethylcarboline carboxylate
DMCTC dimethylchlortetracycline
DMD Doctor of Dental Medicine; Duchenne muscular dystrophy
DMDT dimethoxydiphenyl trichloroethane; methoxychlor (Marlate)
DME Director of Medical Education; Dulbecco's modified Eagle's (medium)
DMF In dentistry, formula representing a number of decayed, missing, and filled teeth (with reference to permanent teeth)
DMFT decayed, missing, and filled permanent teeth
DMGBL dimethyl-gamma-butyrolactone
DMHS Director Medical & Health Services
DMJ Diploma in Medical Jurisprudence
DMN dorsal motor nucleus (of the vagus)
DMO District Medical Officer; Divisional Medical Officer
DMP dimethylphthalate
DMPA Depo-medroxyprogesterone acetate
DMPE dimethoxyphenyl-ethylamine
DMR Diploma in Medical Radiology; Directorate of Medical Research (Army)
DMRD Diploma in Medical Radio-Diagnosis
DMRE Diploma in Medical Radiology and Electrology
DMRT Diploma in Medical Radio-Therapy
DMS Department of Medicine and Surgery; dermatomyositis; Director of Medical Services (Armed Forces); District Management Team (Brit); Doctor of Medical Science
DMSO dimethyl sulphoxide
DMSS Director of Medical & Sanitary Services
DMT dimethyltryptamine; Doctor of Medical Technology
DMU dimethanolurea; dimethylurocil
DMV Doctor of Veterinary Medicine
DN dibucaine number; dicrotic notch; Diploma in Nursing; Diploma in Nutrition; District Nurse; Doctor of Nursing

D/N dextrose-nitrogen (ratio)

Dn dekanem (10 nems, *q.v.*)

dn decinem (one tenth of a nem, *q.v.*)

DNA deoxyribonucleic acid; did not attend

DNase deoxyribonuclease

DNB dinitrobenzene; Diplomate of the National Board of Medical Examiners

DNBP dinitrobutylphenol

DNC did not come; Disaster Nursing Chairman

DNCB dinitrochlorobenzene

DNE Director of Nursing Education; Doctor of Nursing Education; Group D non-enterococcal streptococci

DNFB dinitrofluorobenzene

DNL Director of Naval Laboratories

DNMS Director of Naval Medical Services

DNO District Nursing Officer

DNOC Dinitro-ortho-cresol

DNP 2-4-dinitrophenyl group; do not publish

DNPM dinitrophenyl-morphine

DNR daunorubicin (daunomycin); do not resuscitate

DNS diaphragm nerve stimulation; Dinoyl sebacate

DNTP diethyl-nitrophenyl thiophosphate

DO diamine oxidase; Diploma in Ophthalmology; Diploma in Osteopathy; dissolved oxygen; disto-occlusal; Doctor of Ophthalmology; Doctor of Optometry; Doctor of Osteopathy; doctor's orders

do *dictum* (L) the same, as before; ditto

DOA dead on arrival

DOAC Dubois oleic albumin complex (bacteriology)

DOAP daunorubicin, vincristine, cytarabine, and prednisone

DOB date of birth; doctor's order book

DObstRCOG Diploma in Obstetrics, of the Royal College of Obstetricians & Gynaecologists

DOC desoxycorticosterone

doc doctor; document

DOCA desoxycorticosterone acetate

DOCG deoxycorticosterone glucoside

DOcSc Doctor of Ocular Science

DOD died of disease; dissolved oxygen deficit

DOE desoxyephedrine hydrochloride; dyspnoea on exertion

DOHyg Diploma in Occupational Hygiene

DOI died of injuries

DOM *see* STP; Department of Medicine; dominance

(-inant)

dom domestic

DOMS Diploma in Ophthalmic Medicine & Surgery; Doctor of Orthopedic Medicine and Surgery

DON Director of Nursing

don *donec* (L) until

donec alv sol fuerit *donec alvus soluta fuerit* (L) until the bowels are opened

DOPA dihydroxy-phenylalanine

dopase dopa oxidase

DOph Doctor of Ophthalmology

DOrth Diploma in Orthodontics (Brit); Diploma in Orthoptics (Brit)

DOS deoxystreptamine; Doctor of Ocular Science; Doctor of Optical Science

dos dosage; *dosis* (L) dose

DOSC Dubois oleic serum complex (bacteriology)

DOSS distal over-shoulder strap

DP deep pulse; degradation products; dementia praecox; dental prosthetics; diffusion pressure; digestible protein; diphosgene; diphosphate; dipropionate; *directione propria* (L) with proper direction; displaced person; distopulpal; Doctor of Pharmacy; donor's plasma

D-P Depo-Provera (medroxyprogesterone acetate)

DPA diphenylamine; dipicolinic acid

DPC direct patient care; desaturated phosphatidylcholine; distal palmar crease

DPD Department of Public Dispensary; diphenamid; Diploma in Public Dentistry

DPDA phosphorodiamidic anhydride

DPF Dental Practitioners' Formulary

DPG diphosphoglycerate

DPGM diphosphoglycerate mutase

DPH Department of Public Health; diphenylhydantoin; Diploma in Public Health; Doctor of Public Health; Doctor of Public Hygiene

DPh Doctor of Philosophy

DPhC Doctor of Pharmaceutical Chemistry

DPhc Doctor of Pharmacology

DPhEd Doctor of Public Health Education

DPHEng Doctor of Public Health Engineering

DPHN Doctor of Public Health Nursing

DPhys Diploma in Physiotherapy

DPhysMed Diploma in Physical Medicine

DPIF Drug Product Information File

DPL   dipalmitoyl lecithin; distopulpolingual

DPLa   distopulpolabial

DPM   Diploma in Psychological Medicine; discontinue previous medication; Doctor of Physical Medicine; Doctor of Preventative Medicine; Doctor of Podiatric Medicine; Doctor of Psychiatric Medicine

Dr   Doctor

dr   dorsal root (of spinal nerves); drachm (dram); dressing

DRACOG   Diploma of Royal Australian College of Obstetricians and Gynaecologists

DRACR   Diploma of Royal Australasian College of Radiologists

dr ap   drachm apothecaries' weight

DRCOG   Diploma of the Royal College of Obstetricians and Gynaecologists

DRCPath   Diploma of the Royal College of Pathologists

DRF   daily replacement factor (of lymphocytes); Deafness Research Foundation

DRG   diagnostic related group; dorsal respiratory group (of neurons); dorsal root ganglion

DrHyg   Doctor of Hygiene

dRib   deoxyribose

DRIC   Dental Research Information Center

DRME   Division of Research in Medical Education

Dr Med   Doctor of Medicine

DrMT   Doctor of Mechanotherapy

DRnt   diagnostic roentgenology

DRO   Disablement Resettlement Officer (Brit)

DRP   *Deutsches Reichs-Patent* (German patent)

DrPH   Doctor of Public Health; Doctor of Public Hygiene

DrPHHy   Doctor of Public Health and Hygiene

DRQ   discomfort relief quotient

DRS   drowsiness

drsg   dressing

DRVO   Deputy Regional Veterinary Officer

DS   dead-air space; density (optical) standard; Dental Surgery; Dermatology and Syphilology; dilute strength (of solutions); dioptric strength; Disaster Services (Red Cross); disseminated sclerosis; dissolved solids; Doctor of Science; donor's serum; double-stranded (DNA); double strength; Down's syndrome; drug store

D/S   dextrose and saline; dominance and submission

D-5-S   dextrose (5%) in saline

DSAS   discrete subaortic stenosis
DSB   Dictionary of Scientific Biography; Drug Supervising Body
DSBL   disabled
DSC   disodium cromoglycate; Doctor of Surgical Chiropody
DSc   Doctor of Science
DSCS   disodium cromoglycate
DSD   dry sterile dressing
DSE   Doctor of Sanitary Engineering
DSI   Down's Syndrome International
DSIM   Doctor of Science in Industrial Medicine
DSIP   delta sleep-inducing peptide
dslv   dissolved
DSM   Diagnostic and Statistical Manual of Mental Disorders; Diploma in Social Medicine (Brit)
dsRNA   double-stranded ribonucleic acid
DSS   dioctyl sodium sulphosuccinate (docusate sodium)
DSSc   Diploma in Sanitary Science
DST   daylight saving time; desensitization test; dexamethasone suppression test; dihydrostreptomycin
DSUH   direct suggestion under hypnosis
DSur   Doctor of Surgery
DT   delirium tremens; Dental Technician; diphtheria-tetanus; dispensing tablet; distance test; duration of tetany
D/T   deaths: total ratio
DTCD   Diploma in Tuberculosis & Chest Diseases
DTCH   Diploma in Tropical Child Health
DTD   Diploma in Tuberculous Diseases (Brit)
dtd   *datur talis dosis* (L) give of such a dose
dtdNo iv   *dentur tales doses No. iv* (L) let four such doses be given
DTH   delayed-type hypersensitivity; Diploma in Tropical Hygiene
DTIC   5-(3,   3-dimethyl-1-triazino)imidazole-4-carboxamide (dacarbazine)
DTM   Diploma in Tropical Medicine
DTMA   desoxycorticosterone trimethylacetate
DTM&H   Diplomate of Tropical Medicine and Hygiene
DTN   diphtheria toxin, normal
DTNB   dithionitrobenzene
DTP   diphtheria, tetanus, pertussis; distal tingling on percussion
DTPH   Diploma in Tropical Public Health

DTR deep tendon reflex

DTS dense tubular system

DTT diphtheria-tetanus toxoid; dithiothreitol

DT-VAC diphtheria tetanus vaccine

DTVM Diploma in Tropical Veterinary Medicine

DU diagnosis undetermined; density (optical) unknown; dog unit (with reference to adrenal cortical hormones); duodenal ulcer

DUB dysfunctional uterine bleeding

dulc *dulcis* (L) sweet

dUMP deoxyuridine monophosphate

duod duodenum

dup duplicate

dur *duris* (L) hard

dur dol *durante dolore* (L) while the pain lasts

DV dependent variable; dilute volume (of solutions); distemper virus; divorced; domiciliary visit; double vision

dv double vibrations

D&V diarrhoea and vomiting

DVA duration of voluntary apnoea (test)

DVCC Disease Vector Control Center

DV&D Diploma in Venereology and Dermatology

DVDALV double vessel disease with an abnormal left ventricle

DVE duck virus enteritis

DVH Diploma in Veterinary Hygiene; Division for the Visually Handicapped

DVM Doctor of Veterinary Medicine

DVMS Doctor of Veterinary Medicine and Surgery

DVO Divisional Veterinary Office

DVOP Disabled Veterans Outreach Program

DVR Department of Vocational Rehabilitation; Doctor of Veterinary Radiology

DVS Doctor of Veterinary Science; Doctor of Veterinary Surgery

DVSc Doctor of Veterinary Science

DVSM Diploma of Veterinary State Medicine

DVT deep venous thrombosis

DW distilled water

D/W dextrose in water

D-5-W dextrose (5%) in water

DWA died from woulds resulting from action with the enemy

DWD died with disease

DWS Disaster Warning System

dwt pennyweight
Dx diagnosis
DXM dexamethasone (test for adrenocortical function)
DXR deep X-ray
DXRT deep X-ray therapy
DXT deep X-ray therapy; dextrose
dyn dyne
DZ dizygotic; dizziness

E

E electrode potential; electromotive force; emmetropia; endoplasm; energy; enzyme; erythrocyte; *Escherichia;* esophagus; ester; estradiol; ethyl; experiment(-al); expired gas; extralymphatic; eye
e electric charge; electron; *ex* (L) from
ε epsilon
E_0 electric affinity
4E four plus oedema
EA educational age; electric affinity; endocardiographic amplifier; Endometriosis Association; erythrocyte antibody; estivoautumnal (malaria)
ea each
EAA Epilepsy Association of America; essential amino acid; extrinsic allergic alveolitis
EAB Ethics Advisory Board (HHS)
EAC erythrocyte antibody complement; external auditory canal
EACA ε-aminocaproic acid
EACD eczematous allergic contact dermatitis
ead *eadem* (L) the same
EAE experimental allergic encephalomyelitis; experimental autoimmune encephalitis
EAHF eczema, asthma, and hay fever
EAI Emphysema Anonymous, Inc.
EAM external acoustic meatus
EAMG experimental autoimmune myasthenia gravis
EAN experimental allergic neuritis
EAP electroacupuncture; epiallopregnanolone; erythrocyte acid phosphatase
EaR *Entartungs-Reaktion* (Ger) reaction of degeneration (*see* RD)

EAT electroaerosol therapy; experimental autoimmune thymitis

EATC Ehrlich ascites tumour cell

EB elementary body; epidermolysis bullosa; Epstein-Barr (virus); estradiol benzoate

EBD epidermolysis bullosa dystrophia

EBDD epidermolysis bullosa dystrophia dominant

EBDR epidermolysis bullosa dystrophia recessive

EBF erythroblastosis fetalis

EBI emetine bismuth iodide

EBK embryonic bovine kidney

EBM expressed breast milk

E/BOD electrolytic biological oxygen demand

EBP estradiol-binding protein

EBS electric brain stimulator; Emergency Bed Service; epidermolysis bullosa simplex

EBV Epstein-Barr virus

EC electrochemical; electron capture; enteric coated (with reference to tablets); entering complaint; enterochromaffin cells; Enzyme Commission; epidermal cell; expiratory centre; extracellular; eyes closed

E/C estrogen to creatinine (ratio)

E-C ether-chloroform (mixture)

ECA ethylcarboxylate adenosine

ECBO enteric cytopathogenic bovine orphan (virus)

ECC electrocorticogram; emergency cardiac care

ECD electron capture detector; endocardial cushion defect

ECDO enteric cytopathic dog orphan (virus)

ECF Extended Care Facility; extracellular fluid

ECFMG Educational Commission for Foreign Medical Graduates

ECFMS Educational Council for Foreign Medical Students

ECG electrocardiogram(-ograph)

ECGF endothelial cell growth factor

ECHO echoencephalogram (sonoencephalon); enterocytopathogenic human orphan (virus)

ECI extracorporeal irradiation

Eclec eclectic

ECM embryo chicken muscle; extracellular material

ECMO enteric cytopathic monkey orphan (virus); extracorporeal membrane oxygenation

ECMP entero-coated microspheres of pancrelipase

ECOG Eastern Cooperative Oncology Group

E coli *Escherichia coli*
ECP *Escherichia coli* polypeptides; estradiol cyclopentane-propionate; free cytoporphyrin in erythrocytes
ECPO enteric cytopathogenic porcine orphan (virus)
ECPOG electrochemical potential gradient
ECS electroconvulsive shock; elective cosmetic surgery
ECSO enteric cytopathic swine orphan (virus)
ECT electroconvulsive (electroshock) therapy; enteric coated tablet
ECV extracellular volume
ED effective dose; electrodialysis; Emergency Department; Entner-Doudoroff (metabolic pathway); enzymatic deficiencies; epidural; erythema dose; ethynodiol; ethyl dichlorarsine; extra-low dispersion
Ed editor
ed edition
ED$_{50}$ median effective dose
EDB early dry breakfast
EDC Emergency Decontamination Center; expected date of confinement
EDD enzyme-digested delta (endotoxin); expected date of delivery
edent edentulous
E-diol estradiol
EDL end-diastolic length
ED/LD emotionally disturbed/learning disabled
EDM early diastolic murmur
EDN electrodesiccation
EDNA Emergency Department Nurses Association
EDP electron dense particles; electronic data processing; end diastolic pressure; epatite degenerative-proliferative (hepatic virus)
EDR effective direct radiation; electrodermal response; electrodialysis with reversed polarity
EDS Ehlers-Danlos Syndrome
EDTA ethylenediaminetetra-acetic acid (edetic acid; edathamil)
EDV end diastolic volume
EDWTH end-diastolic wall thickness
EDx electrodiagnosis
EDXA energy-dispersive X-ray analysis
EE embryo extract; enterobacteriaceae enrichment (broth); equine encephalitis; eye and ear
E-E erythematous-edematous (reaction)

EE3ME ethinyloestradiol-3-methyl ether (mestranol)
EEE eastern equine encephalitis
EEG electroencephalograph(-gram)
EENT eyes, ears, nose and throat
EEPI extraretinal eye position information
EES erythromycin ethylsuccinate; ethyl ethanesulphate
EF edema factor; ejection fraction; Emergency Facilities; eosinophilic fasciitis; equivalent focus; extra fine; extrinsic factor
EFA Epilepsy Foundation of America; essential fatty acids
EFE endocardial fibro-elastosis
EFF efficiency
eff effects; efferent
effect effective
effer efferent
EFL effective focal length
EFM electronic fetal monitoring
EFP effective filtration pressure
EFR effective filtration rate
eg *exempli gratio* (L) for example
EGD esophagogastroduodenoscopy
EGDF embryonic growth and development factor
EGF epidermal growth factor
EGTA esophageal gastric tube airway; ethylene glycol tetra-acetic acid
EH enlarged heart; essential hypertension
E&H environment and heredity (psychology)
eH oxidation-reduction potential
EHA Emotional Health Anonymous; Environmental Health Agency
EHAA epidermic hepatitis-associated antigen
EHBF extrahepatic blood flow
EHC enterohepatic circulation; enterohepatic clearance; extended health care
EHD epizootic haemorrhagic disease (of poultry)
EHL effective half-life (of radioactive substances); Environmental Health Laboratory
EHME Employee Health Maintenance Examination
EHP di-(2-ethylhexyl) hydrogen phosphate; extra high potency
EHPAC Emergency Health Preparedness Advisory Committee
EHPT Eddy hot plate test
EHSDS Experimental Health Service Delivery System

EHV   electric heat vector; equine herpes virus
EI   electrolyte imbalance
EIA   electroimmunoassay
EIB   exercise-induced bronchiospasm
EIC   elastase inhibitory capacity
eIF   erythrocyte initiation factor
EIPS   endogenous inhibitor of prostaglandin synthase
EIRnv   extra incidence rate in non-vaccinated groups
EIRv   extra incidence rate in vaccinated groups
EIS   Epidemic Intelligence Service (CDC); Environmental Impact Statement
EIT   erythroid iron turnover
EJ   elbow jerk
EJP   excitatory junction potential
ejusd   *ejusdem* (L) of the same
EKG   electrocardiograph(-gram) (*see* ECG); epidemic keratoconjunctivitis
EKY   electrokymograph(-gram)
EL   early latent; exercise limit
ELB   early light breakfast
elec   electric(al); electricity
elect   *electuarium* (L) electuary
elem   elementary
elev   elevator(-ation)(-ate)
ELH   egg-laying hormone
ELIEDA   enzyme-linked immuno-electro-diffusion assay
ELISA   enzyme-linked immunoadsorbent assay
elix   *elixir* (L) elixir
ELP   endogenous limbic potential
ELSS   Emergency Life Support System
EM   electron microscope(-scopy); electrophoretic mobility; Emergency Medicine; emotionally disturbed
E-M   Embden-Meyerhof (glycolytic pathway)
E&M   endocrine and metabolism
Em   emmetropia (normal vision)
EMA   Emergency Assistant(-ance)
Emb   embryology
EMB   engineering in medicine and biology; eosin-methylene blue (agar); ethambutol; explosive mental behaviour
EMBASE   Excerpta Medica database
EMBL   European Molecular Biology Laboratory
embryol   embryology
EMC   Emergency Medical Care; encephalomyocarditis
EMC&R   Emergency Medical Care and Rescue

EMCRO Experimental Medical Care Review Organization

EMD esophageal mobility disorder

emend *emendatis* (L) emended

emer emergency

EMF electromotive force; Emergency Medicine Foundation; endomyocardial fibrosis; erythrocyte maturation factor

EMG electromyograph(-gram); exomphalos, macroglossia and giantism (syndrome); eye movement gauge

EMGORS electromyogram sensors

EMI Emergency Medical Information

EMIC emergency maternity and infant care

EMIT enzyme multiplied immunoassay technique

EMJH Ellinghausen, McCullough, Johnson, Harris (medium)

EMMA eye-movement measuring apparatus

EMO Epstein and Macintosh, Oxford (ether inhaler and Oxford bellows)

emot emotion(al)

emp *emplastrum* (L) a plaster; *ex modo prescripto* (L) after the manner prescribed, as directed

emp vesic *emplastrum vesicatorium* (L) a blistering plaster

EMRA Emergency Medicine Residents Association

EMS early morning specimen; Electronic Medical Service; Emergency Medical Service

EMSS Emergency Medical Service System

EMT Emergency Medical Tag; Emergency Medical Technician; Emergency Medical Treatment

emu electromagnetic unit

emuls *emulsio* (L) an emulsion

EN enrolled nurse; erythema nodosum

en enema; ethylene diamine (in chemical formulas)

ENA extractable nuclear antigens

Endo endodontics

Endocrin endocrinology

enem enema

ENG electronystagmograph(-gram)

Eng England

ENP ethyl-*p*-nitrophenylthiobenzene-phosphate

ENR eosinophilic nonallergic rhinitis; extrathyroidal neck radioactivity

ENT ears, nose and throat

Entom entomology

ENU ethylnitrosourea

environ environment(al)

EOA examination, opinion, and advice

E of M error of measurement

EOG electro-oculogram

EOL end of life

EOM extraocular movement; extraocular muscles

EOMA emergency oxygen mask assembly

Eos eosinophil(s)

Eosins eosinophils

EOU epidemic observation unit

EP ectopic pregnancy; edible portion (of a food); electrophoresis; Emergency Procedures; endogenous pyrogen; endpoint; enzyme product; epithelial(-ioid); erythrophagocytosis; erythropoietic porphyria; erythropoietin; evoked potential; extreme pressure; protoporphyrin (free in erythrocytes)

EPA eicosapentaenoic acid; erect posterior-anterior; Environmental Protection Agency (US)

EPC epilepsy partialis continua; external pneumatic compression

EPDML epidemiology(-ological)(-ologist)

EPEC enteropathogenic *Escherichia coli*

EPF endothelial proliferating factor; exophthalmos-producing factor

EPG eggs per gram (parasitology); electropneumogram (-graph)

EPI epithelium(-ial); evoked potential index

epid epidemic

Epil epilepsy(-leptic)

epineph epinephrine

epis episiotomy

epistom *epistomium* (L) a stopper

epith epithelium(-ial)

EMP energy-protein malnutrition

EPP end-plate potential; erythropoietic protoporphyria

EPPS Edwards Personal Preference Schedule

EPR electrophrenic respiration

EPS elastosis performans serpiginosa; exophthalmos-producing substance (of anterior pituitary); extrapyramidal symptoms

ep's epithelial cells

EPSP excitatory post-synaptic potential

EPT early pregnancy test

EPTS existed prior to services

EQ 82

EQ educational quotient; encephalization quotient

eq equation; equivalent

equip equipment

equiv equivalent

ER emergency room; endoplasmic reticulum; environmental resistance; equivalent roentgen (unit); estrogen receptor; evoked response; extended release; external resistance

Er erythrocyte

ERA electrical response activity; Electroshock Research Association; evoked response audiometry

ERBF effective renal blood flow

ERC ECHO-rhino-coryza (viruses); endoscopic retrograde cholangiography; erythropoietin responsive cell

ERCP endoscopic retrograde cholangiopancreatographic (examination)

ERD evoked response detector

ERDA Energy Research and Development Administration

ERF Education and Research Foundation (AMA); Eye Research Foundation

ERG electroretinogram(-graph)

ERIA electroradio-immuno assay

ERM electrochemical relaxation methods

ERP effective refractory period; endoscopic retrograde pancreatography; estrogen receptor protein

ERPF effective renal plasma flow

ERSP event-related slow-brain potential

ERT estrogen replacement therapy

ERV expiratory reserve volume

ERY erysipelas

Ery *Erysipelothrix*

ES ejection sound; elastic suspensor; electrical stimulus; electroshock; Emergency Service; enema saponis; enzyme substrate

ESA Electrolysis Society of America

ESB electrical stimulation to brain

ESC erythropoietin-sensitive stem cells

Esch *Escherichia*

ESCN electrolyte and steroid-produced cardiopathy characterized by necrosis

ESE *electrostatische Einheit* (Ger) electrostatic unit

ESF erythropoietic stimulating factor (*see* EMF)

ESL end-systolic length

ESN educationally subnormal; estrogen-stimulated

neurophysin

esoph esophagus

ESP end systolic pressure; evoked synaptic potential; extrasensory perception

esp especial(ly)

ESR electron spin resonance; erythrocyte sedimentation rate

ESRD end stage renal disease

ESS erythrocyte sensitizing substance

EST electroshock therapy; esterase

est estimated

esth esthetic

est wt estimated weight

ESU Electrosurgical Unit

esu electrostatic unit

E sub excitor substance

ESV end-systolic volume; esophageal valve

ET educational therapy; endotracheal tube; Enterostomal Therapist; essential thrombocythemia; esotropia for distance; extraterrestrial

ET-3 erythrocyte tri-iodothyronine

Et ethyl

et al *et alibi* (L) and elsewhere; *et alii* (L) and others

ETC estimated time of conception

etc *et cetera* (L) and others of the like kind; and so forth

ETEC enterotoxigenic *Escherichia coli*

ETF electron-transferring flavoprotein

eth ether

ETIO etiocholandone

etiol etiology

ETO estimated time of ovulation

EtOH ethyl alcohol

ETP electron transport particle

ETR effective thyroxine ratio

et seq *et sequentes* (L) and those that follow

ETT exercise tolerance test

ETU Emergency and Trauma Unit; Emergency Treatment Unit

EU Entropy Unit; Enzyme Unit

EUA examination under anaesthesia

EUROTOX European Committee on Chronic Toxicity Hazards

EUS external urethral sphincter

EUV extreme ultraviolet laser

EV Emergency Vehicle; extravascular

eV electron volt (SI)
ev electron volt; eversion
EVA ethyl violet azide (broth); ethylene vinyl acetate
evac evacuated
eval evaluate(-tion)
evap evaporated
ever eversion
EVP evoked visual potential
EVR evoked response
EW Emergency Ward
EWL evaporative water loss
ex exaggerated; examined; example; exercise
ex aff *ex affinis* (L) of affinity
exag exaggerated
exam examination
exc except(ed)
exer exercise
ex gr *ex grupa* (L) of the group of
exhib *exhibeatur* (L) let it be given
exp expecting(ed); experiment(al); expired
expect *expectorant* (L) expectorant
exper experiment(al)
ExPGN extracapillary proliferative glomerular nephritis
expir expiration(-atory)
expt expected; experimental
exptl experimental
EXREM external radiation dose
Ext extraction (dentistry)
ext *extend* (L) spread; extension; extensor; external; *extractum* (L) extract; extremity
extd extended; extracted
ext fl fluid extract
ext rot external rotation
exx examples
EY egg yolk
EYA egg yolk-pyruvate-tellurite-glycine agar
Ez eczema

F

F facies; factor; Fahrenheit (temperature scale); failure; family; farad (SI); fasting (test); father; fats; Fellow;

female; feminine; fertility; fertility factor; fetal; fibrous (with reference to proteins); field of vision; filament; fine; finger; flow (of blood); fluorine; focal length; foil (dentistry); formula(ry); fractional (with reference to fractional composition of gases); fracture; free; French (catheter size); frontal; full (with reference to diet); function

f *fac, fiat, fiant* (L) make, let it be made, let them be made; farad; fluid; focal; *forma* (L) form; frequency; from

F₁ first filial generation

F₂ second filial generation; zinc oxide-eugenol cement (dentistry)

f-12 freon

FA Families Anonymous; fatty acid; febrile antigens; femoral artery; fibrosing alveolitis; field ambulance; filterable agent; first aid; fluorescent antibody; folic acid; fortified aqueous (with reference to solutions); Freund's adjuvant; functional activities

FAA sol formalin, acetic, alcohol solution (a fixative)

FAB antigen-binding fragments; functional arm brace

Fab antigen-binding fragment of an antigen

FAC free available chlorine

Fac factor

FACA Fellow of the American College of Anesthetists; Fellow of the American College of Angiology; Fellow of the American College of Apothecaries

FACAl Fellow of the American College of Allergists

FACC Fellow of the American College of Cardiologists

FACCP Fellow of the American College of Chest Physicians

FACD Fellow of the American College of Dentists

FACFP Fellow of the American College of Family Physicians

FACFS Fellow of the American College of Foot Surgeons

FACG Fellow of the American College of Gastroenterology

FACHA Fellow of the American College of Health Administrators

FACMTA Federal Advisory Council on Medical Training Aids

FACNHA Foundation of American College of Nursing Home Administrators

FACO Fellow of the American College of Otolaryngology

FACOG Fellow of the American College of Obstetricians and Gynecologists

FACOSH Federal Advisory Committee on Occupational Safety and Health

FACP Fellow of the American College of Physicians

FACPM Fellow of the American College of Preventative Medicine

FACR Fellow of the American College of Radiology

FACS Fellow of the American College of Surgeons; fluorescence-activated cell sorter

FACSM Fellow of the American College of Sports Medicine

FACT Flanagan Aptitude Classification Test

FAD familial autonomic dysfunction; fetal activity-acceleration determination; flavine adenine dinucleotide

FADH₂ flavine adenine dinucleotide (reduced form)

FADN flavine adenine dinucleotide

FAH Federation of American Hospitals

Fahr Fahrenheit

FAI First Aid Instructor

FAIT First Aid Instructor Trainer

FALG fowl antimouse lymphocyte globulin

Fam family

FAMA Fellow of the American Medical Association

FAME fatty acid methyl ester

Fam per par familial periodic paralysis

Fam phys family physician

FANA fluorescent antinuclear antibody

FANPT Freeman Anxiety Neurosis and Psychosomatic Test

FANS Fellow of the American Neurological Society

FANY First Aid Nursing Yeomanry (Brit)

FAO Food and Agricultural Organization (of the United Nations)

FAPA Fellow of the American Psychiatric Association; Fellow of the American Psychoanalytical Association

FAPHA Fellow of the American Public Health Association

FAR flight aptitude rating

far faradic

FARE Federation of Alcoholic Rehabilitation Establishments (Brit)

FAS Federation of American Scientists; fetal alcohol syndrome

FASC Free-standing Ambulatory Surgical Centre

fasc *fasciculus* (L) bundle

FASEB Federation of American Societies for Experimental Biology

FAST fluorescent antibody staining technique

FAT fluorescent antibody technique; Food Awareness Training

FB feedback; fibreoptic bronchoscopy; finger breadth; foreign body

FBA Fellow of the British Academy

FBCOD foreign body cornea right eye

FBCOS foreign body cornea left eye

FBF forearm blood flow

FBG fibrinogen

FBH familial benign hypocalciuric hypercalcaemia

FBI flossing, brushing and irrigation (dentistry)

FBL follicular basal lamina

FBN Federal Bureau of Narcotics

FBPsS Fellow of the British Psychological Society

FBS fasting blood sugar; feedback signal; feedback system; fetal bovine serum

FC fast component (of an axon); faecal coli (broth); Foley catheter

Fc crystallizable fragment (of Ig)

fc foot candle

FCA Freund's complete adjuvant

FCAP Fellow of the College of American Pathologists

FCC Federal Communications Commission

FCCP Fellow of the American College of Chest Physicians

FCD faecal collection device

FChS Fellow of the Society of Chiropodists

fcly face lying

FCMS Fellow of the College of Medicine and Surgery

FCMW Foundation for Child Mental Welfare

FCO Fellow of the College of Osteopathy

FCP final common pathway (neurology)

FCPS Fellow of the College of Physicians and Surgeons

FCPSA(SoAf) Fellow of the College of Physicians and Surgeons, S Africa

FCRA faecal collection receptacle assembly; Fellow of the College of Radiologists of Australasia

FCRC Frederick Cancer Research Center

FCS faecal containment system; feedback control

system; Fellow of the Chemical Society; fetal calf serum

FCSP Fellow of the Chartered Society of Physiotherapy

FCST Fellow of the College of Speech Therapists

FD familial dysautonomia; fan douche; fatal dose; focal distance; forceps delivery; freeze-dried

FD$_{50}$ median fatal dose (that fatal to 50% of test subjects)

FDA Food and Drug Administration; *frontodextra-anterior* (L) right frontoanterior (position of fetus)

FD&C Food, Drug and Cosmetic (Act)

FDCPA Food, Drug and Consumer Product Agency (HHS)

FDD Food and Drugs Directorate (Canada)

FDDC ferric dimethyldithiocarbonate

FDF fast death factor

FDG fluorodeoxyglucose

fdg feeding

FDI Fédération Dentaire Internationale

FDIU fetal death in utero

FDNB fluorodinitrobenzene

FDO Fleet Dental Officer

FDP fibrin degradation product; *frontodextra posterior* (L) right frontoposterior (position of fetus); fructose diphosphate

fdp/Fdp fibrin/fibrinogen degradation products

FDS Fellow in Dental Surgery

FDSRCSEng Fellow in Dental Surgery of the Royal College of Surgeons of England

FDT *frontodextra transversa* (L) right frontotransverse (position of fetus)

FDV Friend disease virus

FE faecal emesis; faecal energy; fetal erythroblastosis; fluid extract

Fe *ferrum* (L) iron

^{59}Fe radioactive iron

feb *febus* (L) fever

feb dur *febre durante* (L) while the fever lasts

FEBP fetoneonatal estrogen-binding protein

FECG fetal electrocardiogram

FECT fibroelastic connective tissue

Fed federal; federation

Fed spec federal specifications

FEE forced equilibrating expiration

FEKG fetal electrocardiogram

Fel Fellow

FEM *femoris* (L) thigh

fem female; feminine

Fem intern *femoribus internus* (L) at the inner side of the thighs

FEP fluorinated ethylene propylene; free erythrocyte protoporphyrin

Fer *ferrum* (L) iron

fertd fertilized

FEUO for external use only

ferv *fervens* (L) boiling

FEV₁ forced expiratory volume in one second

FF fat free; fertility factor; filtration fraction; fixing fluid; follicular fluid; foster father; fresh frozen

ff following; force fluid

FFA Fellow of the Faculty of Anaesthetists; free fatty acid

FFAP free fatty acid phase

FFARCS Fellow of the Faculty of Anaesthetists, RCS

FFC free from chlorine

FFCM Fellow of Faculty of Community Medicine

FFD Fellow in the Faculty of Dentistry; focus film distance (X-ray)

FFDCA Federal Food, Drug, and Cosmetic Act

FFDSRCS Fellow of the Faculty of Dental Surgery Royal College of Surgeons

FFDW fat-free dry weight

FFHom Fellow of the Faculty of Homeopathy

FFI free from infection

FFIT fluorescent focus inhibition test

FFOM Fellow of Faculty of Occupational Medicine

FFP fresh frozen plasma

FFR Fellow of the Faculty of Radiologists

FFS fat-free solids; fat-free supper

FFT flicker fusion threshold

FFU focus-forming unit

FFWW fat-free wet weight

F-G Feeley-Gorman (agar)

FGS focal glomerulosclerosis

FH familial hypercholesterolaemia; family history; fetal heart; Frankfort horizontal (plane of skull)

fh *fiat haustus* (L) let a draught be made

FHA Fellow of the Institute of Hospital Administrators

FHF fulminant hepatic failure

FHH fetal heart heard

FHIP Family Health Insurance Plan

FHNH fetal heart not heard

FHR familial hypophosphataemic rickets; fetal heart rate

FHS fetal heart sounds; fetal hydantoin syndrome

FHT fetal heart tone

FI fixed internal (reinforcement)

FIA Freund's incomplete adjuvant

FIAT Field Information Agency, Technical (US Reports)

FIB Fellow of the Institute of Biology (Brit); fibrin; fibrinogen; fibrositis; fibula

fibrill fibrillation

FIC Fellow of the Institute of Chemistry

FICA Federal Insurance Contribution Act (Social Security)

FICD Fellow of the Institute of Canadian Dentists; Fellow of the International College of Dentists

FICS Fellow of the International College of Surgeons

FID flame ionization detector

FIF feedback inhibition factor; fibroblast interferon

FIFRA Federal Insecticide, Fungicide and Rodenticide Act

fig figuratively; figure

FIGLU formiminoglutamic acid

FIH fat-induced hyperglycaemia

fil filamentous

filt *filtra* (L) filter

FIM field ion microscope(-scopy)

FIMF International Federation of Physical Medicine

FIMLT Fellow of the Institute of Medical Laboratory Technology

FIN fine intestinal needle

FInstSP Fellow of the Institute of Sewage Purification

FIO$_2$ fractional inspiratory oxygen

FIR far infrared

fist fistula

FIUO for internal use only

F-J Fisher-John (melting point method)

FJRM full joint range of movement

FL fluorescence(-ent); focal length; frontal lobe (of the brain)

fL foot-lambert

fl flexion; *fluidium* (L) fluid

FLA *frontolaeva anterior* (L) left fronto-anterior (position of fetus)

fla *fiat lege artis* (L) let it be done according to rule

flac flaccid
flav *flavus* (L) yellow
FLC Friend leukaemia cells
fld fluid
fl dr fluid drachm (dram)
fldxt *fluidextractum* (L) fluid extract
FLEX Federal Licensing Examination
flex flexion, flexor
FLK funny looking kid (paediatrics)
flocc flocculation
flor *flores* (L) flowers
fl oz fluid ounce
FLP *frontolaeva posterior* (L) left frontoposterior (position of fetus)
FLS Fellow of the Linnean Society; fibrous long spacing (collagen)
FLSP fluorescein-labelled serum protein
FLT *frontolaeva transversa* (L) left frontotransverse (position of fetus)
fluor fluoroscopy; fluorescent
fluores fluorescent
FLV Friend leukaemia virus
FM feedback mechanism; flavin mononucleotide; forensic medicine; formerly married; foster mother; frequency modulation; fusobacteria micro-organisms
fm *fiat mistura* (L) make a mixture
FMB full maternal behaviour
FMC Flight Medicine Clinic; Foundation for Medical Care
FMCA Forensic Medicine Consultant-Advisor
FMD foot and mouth disease
FMDV foot-and-mouth disease virus
FME full mouth extraction
FMF familial Mediterranean fever; fetal movement felt
FMG Foreign Medical Graduates
FMH fat-mobilizing hormone
FMN flavin mononucleotide
FMNH flavin mononucleotide (reduced form)
FMO Fleet Medical Officer; Flight Medical Officer
FMP first menstrual period
FMS fat-mobilizing substance; Fellow of the Medical Society; full mouth series
FMX full mouth radiography (dentistry)
F-N finger to nose
FNA fine needle aspiration

Fneg false negative
FNP Family Nurse Practitioner
f-number focal length (of a lens)
FO foramen ovale; frontooccipital
FOA Federation of Orthodontic Associations
FOB faecal occult blood; feet out of bed; fibreoptic bronchoscopy
fol *folium* (L) a leaf; following
FOPR full outpatient rate
FOR forensic (pathology)
for foreign
form formation; formula
fort *fortis* (L) strong
Found foundation
FP Family Planning; family practice; Family Practitioner; fibrinopeptide; filter paper; flat paper; flavin phosphate (riboflavine 5'-phosphate); flavoprotein; food poisoning; frozen plasma
fp *fiat potio* (L) let a potion be made; foot-pound; forearm pronated; freezing point
FPA Family Planning Association; fibrinopeptide A; filter paper activity
FPB femoral popliteal bypass
FPC Family Planning Clinic; Family Practioner Committee; fish protein concentrate
FPG fluorescence plus Giemsa
FPH$_2$ flavin phosphate (reduced form)
FPHE formalin-treated pyruvaldehyde-stabilized human erythrocytes
f pil *fiant pilulae* (L) let pills be made
f pil xi *fac pilulas xi* (L) make 11 pills
FPM filter paper microscopic (test)
fpm feet per minute
FPO freezing point osmometer
FPRA first-pass radionuclide angiogram
FPS Fellow of the Pathological Society; Fellow of the Pharmaceutical Society
fps feet per second; foot-pound-second
FPV fowl plague virus
FPVB femoral popliteal vein bypass
F&R force and rhythm (of pulse)
FR failure rate (with reference to contraception); fixed ratio; flocculation reaction
Fr French
fr from

FRA fluorescent rabies antibody

FRACDS Fellow of the Royal Australasian College of Dental Surgery

FRCGP Fellow of the Royal Australasian College of General Practitioners

FRACO Fellow of the Royal Australasian College of Ophthalmologists

FRACP Fellow of the Royal Australasian College of Physicians

FRACR Fellow of the Royal Australasian College of Radiologists

FRACS Fellow of the Royal Australasian College of Surgeons

Fract fraction; fracture

fract dos *fracta dosi* (L) in divided doses

FRAI Fellow of the Royal Anthropological Institute

FRANZCP Fellow of the Royal Australian and New Zealand College of Psychiatrists

FRC Federal Radiation Council; frozen red cells; functional residual capacity (of lungs)

FRCD Fellow of the Royal College of Dentists

FRCGP Fellow of the Royal College of General Practitioners

FRCOG Fellow of the Royal College of Obstetricians and Gynaecologists

FRCP Fellow of the Royal College of Physicians

FRCPA Fellow of the Royal College of Pathologists, Australia

FRCPath Fellow of the Royal College of Pathologists

FRCP(C) Fellow of the Royal College of Physicians of Canada

FRCPE Fellow of the Royal College of Physicians of Edinburgh

FRCP(Glasg) Fellow of the Royal College of Physicians and Surgeons of Glasgow *qua* Physician

FRCPI Fellow of the Royal College of Physicians of Ireland

FRCPsych Fellow of the Royal College of Psychiatrists

FRCS Fellow of the Royal College of Surgeons

FRCS(C) Fellow of the Royal College of Surgeons of Canada

FRCSEd Fellow of the Royal College of Surgeons of Edinburgh

FRCSEng Fellow of the Royal College of Surgeons of England

FRCS(Glasg) Fellow of the Royal College of Physicians and Surgeons of Glasgow *qua* Surgeon

FRCSI Fellow of the Royal College of Surgeons in Ireland

FRCVS Fellow of the Royal College of Veterinary Surgeons

FREIR Federal Research on Biological and Health Effects of Ionizing Radiation

frem *fremitus vocalis* (L) vocal fremitus

freq frequency(-ent)

FRES Fellow of the Royal Entomological Society

FRF Fertility Research Foundation; follicle-stimulating hormone releasing factor

FRH follicle-stimulating hormone-releasing hormone

frict friction

Fried test Friedman test (for pregnancy)

frig *frigidus* (L) cold

FRIPHH Fellow of the Royal Institute of Public Health & Hygiene

FRJM full range joint movement

FRMedSoc Fellow of the Royal Medical Society

FRMS Fellow of the Royal Microscopical Society

FROM full range of movement

FRS Fellow of the Royal Society; ferredoxin-reducing substance

FRSC Fellow of the Royal Society of Chemistry

FRSE Fellow of the Royal Society of Edinburgh

FRSH Fellow of the Royal Society of Health

FRT Family Relations Test; full recovery time

fru fructose

frust *frustillatum* (L) in small pieces

FS factor of safety; forearm supinated; fracture, simple; frozen section; full and soft (diet)

fsa *fiat secundum artem* (L) let it be done skilfully

fsar *fiat secundum artem reglas* (L) let it be made according to the rules of the art

FSBT Fowler single breath test

FSC Food Standards Committee (of Ministry of Agriculture, Fisheries, and Food) (UK)

FSD focus skin distance (X-ray)

FSF fibrin stabilizing factor (XIII)

FSGS focal segmental glomerulosclerosis

FSH fascioscapulohumeral; follicle-stimulating hormone

FSHRF follicle-stimulating hormone releasing factor

FSHRH follicle-stimulating hormone releasing hormone

FSI Food Sanitation Institute
FSIA foot shock-induced analgesia
FSMB Federation of State Medical Boards (US)
FSP fibrin split products
FSR Fellow of the Society of Radiographers
FSR-3 isoniazid
FST foam stability test
FSU Family Service Unit
FSV feline fibrosarcoma virus
FT follow through (after Ba meal); formal toxoid; free thyroxine; full term; functional test
ft *fac, fiat, fiant* (L) make, let it be made, let them be made; foot or feet
FTA fluorescent treponemal antibody (test)
FTA-ABS fluorescent treponemal antibody-absorption (test)
FTAT fluorescent treponemal antibody test
FTBD fit to be detained; full term born dead
FTC Federal Trade Commission; frames to come (optometry)
ft c foot candle
ft cataplasm *fiat cataplasma* (L) let a poultice be made
ft cerat *fiat ceratum* (L) let a cerate be made
ft chart vi *fiant chartulae vi* (L) let six powders be made
ft collyr *fiat collyrium* (L) let an eyewash be made
FTD femoral total density
ft emuls *fiat emulsio* (L) let an emulsion be made
ft enem *fiat enema* (L) let an injection (per rectum) be made
ft garg *fiat gargarisma* (L) let a gargle be made
FTI free thyroxine index
ft infus *fiat infusum* (L) let an injection be made (for urethra)
ftL foot-lambert
ft lb foot pound
ft linim *fiat linimentum* (L) let a liniment be made
FTM fluid thioglycolate medium; fractional test meal
ft mas *fiat massa* (L) let a mass be made
ft mass div in pil xiv *fiat massa et divide in pilulae xiv* (L) let 14 pills be made
ft mist *fiat mistura* (L) let a mixture be made
FTND full term normal delivery
ft pil xxiv *fiat pilulae xxiv* (L) let 24 pills be made
ft pulv *fiat pulvis* (L) let a powder be made
ft solut *fiat solutio* (L) let a solution be made

ft suppos *fiat suppositorium* (L) let a suppository be made
FTT failure to thrive; Fever Therapy Technician
ft ung *fiat unguentum* (L) let an ointment be made
FTU fluorescence thiourea
FU faecal urobilinogen; fluorouracil; follow up; fractional urinalysis
Fu Finsen unit (for ultraviolet rays)
FUB functional uterine bleeding
FUDR 2-fluoro-2′-deoxyuridine (floxuridine)
FUM fumarate; fumigate(-ation)
funct function(al)
FUO fever of undetermined origin
FV Friend virus
FVC forced vital capacity
FVR feline viral rhinotracheitis; forearm vascular resistance
f vs *fiat venaesectio* (L) let the patient be bled
FW forced whisper
fw fresh water
FWA Family Welfare Association
FWHM full width at half maximum (tomography)
FWPCA Federal Water Pollution Control Administration
Fx fracture
FY full year
FZS Fellow of the Zoological Society

G

G gap (in cell cycle); gas; gastrin; gauge; gauss; giga (prefix); gingival; globular (with reference to proteins); globulin; glucose; glycine; glycogen; goat (in veterinary medicine); gold inlay (dentistry); gonidial; Grafenberg spot; gram; gravida (pregnant); gravitation constant (Newtonian constant); Greek; green (an indicator colour); gross (leukaemia antigen); guanidine; guanine; guanosine; A unit of force of acceleration (in aviation medicine)
g acceleration due to gravity; gender; gram (SI); group
γ gamma
γG immunoglobulin G
GI, GII, GIII number of previous pregnancies

G-6-P glucose-6-phosphate
GA gastric analysis; general anaesthesia; gentisic acid; gestational age; gingivoaxial; glucuronic acid; gramicidin A; guessed average; gut-associated
Ga gallium; granulocyte agglutination
ga gauge (of needles)
GABA gamma-aminobutyric acid
GADH gastric alcohol dehydrogenase
GADS gonococcal arthritis/dermatitis syndrome
GAL galactosyl
gal galactose; gallon
GALT gut-associated lymphoid tissue
galv galvanic
gang ganglion
gangl ganglion(ic)
garg *gargarismus* (L) gargle
GARP Global Atmospheric Research Program
GAS gastroenterology; general adaptation syndrome; generalized arteriosclerosis
Gastroc gastrocnemius (muscle)
GB gall bladder; goofball (barbiturate pill); Guillain-Barré (syndrome)
GBA gingivobuccoaxial
GBG gonadal steroid-binding globulin
GBH gamma benzene hydrochloride (an isomer of BHC)
GBL glomerular basal lamina
GBM glomerular basement membrane
GBP galactose-binding protein
GBS gall bladder series; glycerine buffered saline; group-B-beta-haemolytic streptococci; Guillain-Barré syndrome
GBSS Gey's balanced salt solution
GC ganglion cells; gas chromatography; Geriatric Care; glucocorticoid; gonococcal infection (gonorrhoea); gonococcus(-al); granulocyte cytotoxic; guanine-cytosine
Gc group-specific component
g-cal gram calorie (small calorie)
GCFT gonorrhoea complement fixation test
GCN giant cerebral neuron
GCS Glasgow Coma Score
GCWM General Conference on Weights and Measures
GD General Dispensary; gonadal dysgenesis
GDB Guide Dogs for the Blind
GDC General Dental Council (Brit)

GDH glutamate dehydrogenase; growth and differentiation hormone (in insects)

GDMO General Duties Medical Officer

GDP guanosine diphosphate

GE gastroenterology(-enteritis); gel electrophoresis; gentamicin

Ge germanium

g-e gravity eliminated

GECC Government Employees' Clinic Centre (Brit)

GEF gonadotrophin enhancing factor

gel gelatin(ous)

gel quav *gelatina quavis* (L) in any kind of jelly

GEN gender; generation; genetics; genital

gen general; *genus* (L) genus

genet genetics

gen et sp nov *genus et species nova* (L) new genus and species

genit genitalia

gen'l general

gen nov *genus novum* (L) new genus

gen proc general procedure

Ger geriatrics; German

Geriat geriatrics

GERL Golgi-associated endoplasmic reticulum lysosomes

Gerontol gerontology(-ologist)

GES glucose electrolyte solution

GEST gestation(al)

GET gastric emptying time

GF germ-free; glass factor (tissue culture); glomerular filtrate; government funded; growth factor

G-F globular-fibrous (with reference to proteins)

gf gram-force

GFAP glial fibrillary acidic protein

G-forces acceleration forces

GFR glomerular filtration rate

GG gamma globulin; glycylglycine

GGE generalized glandular enlargement

GGG *gummi guttae gambiae* (L) gamboge

GH General Hospital; growth (somatotrophic) hormone (of anterior pituitary)

GHAA Group Health Association of America

GHRF growth hormone releasing factor

GHRH growth hormone releasing hormone

GHRIH growth hormone release-inhibiting hormone

GI gastrointestinal; gelatin infusion medium; globin insulin; growth-inhibiting

GIH gastrointestinal hormone

GII gastrointestinal infection

GIK glucose, insulin, and potassium (solution)

ging *gingiva* (L) gum

g-ion gram-ion

GIP gastric inhibitory polypeptide

GIS gastrointestinal series

GIT gastrointestinal tract

GITT glucose insulin tolerance test

GJ gap junctions

Gk Greek

GL glycosphingolipid; greatest length (with reference to embryos)

GL54 athomin

gl gill

g/l grams per litre

GLA gingivolinguoaxial

glac glacial

gland *glandula* (L) a gland; glandular

GLC gas-liquid chromatography

glc glaucoma

GlcA gluconic acid

GLI glicentin (formerly enteroglucagon); glucagon-like immunoreactivity

Gln glutamine

GLO glyoxalase I

Glob globular; globulin

Gltn glomerulo-tubulo-nephritis

Glu glutamic acid; glutamine

Gly glycine

glyc glycerine; *glyceritum* (L) glycerite

GM General Medicine; *grand mal*; monosialoganglioside

gm gram

g/m gallons per minute

GMC General Medical Council (Brit); grivet monkey cell (line)

GMK green monkey kidney (cells)

gm/l grams per litre

gm-m gram-metre

g-mol gram-molecule

GMP guanosine monophosphate

GMS General Medical Services

GM&S general medicine and surgery

GMSC   General Medical Services Committee (Brit)
GMT   Greenwich Mean Time
GMV   gram molecular volume
GMW   gram molecular weight
GN   glomerular nephritis; Graduate Nurse; Gram-negative
G/N   glucose : nitrogen (ratio in urine examination)
Gn   gonadotrophin
GNB   Gram-negative bacilli
GNBM   Gram-negative bacillary meningitis
GNC   general nursing care; General Nursing Council
GNP   Gerontological Nurse Practitioner
GnRF   gonadotrophin-releasing factor
GnRH   gonadotrophin-releasing hormone
GNTP   Graduate Nurse Transition Program
GO   glucose oxidase
G&O   gas and oxygen
GOE   gas, oxygen, ether (in anaesthesia)
GOG   Gynecologic Oncology Group (National Cancer Institute)
GOK   God only knows
GOM   God's own medicine
GOR   general operating room
GOT   glutamic oxalo-acetic transaminase
Gov   governmental
GP   general paralysis; general paresis; general practitioner; genetic prediabetes; geometric progression; globus pallidus; glucose phosphate; Gram-positive; group; guinea pig
GPA   Group Practice Association; guinea pig albumin
GPB   glossopharyngeal breathing
GPBP   guinea pig myelin basic protein
GPD   glucose-6-phosphate dehydrogenase
GPF   granulocytosis-promoting factor
GPGG   guinea pig gamma globulin
GPh   Graduate in Pharmacy
GPI   general paralysis of the insane; glucophosphate isomerase
Gply   gingivoplasty
GPM   general preventive medicine
GPPQ   General Purpose Psychiatric Questionnaire
GPRA   General Practice Reform Association
GPS   guinea pig serum
GPT   glutamic pyruvic transaminase
GpTh   group therapy

GPU guinea-pig unit
GR gamma ray; gastric resection; general research; glutathione reductase
gr gamma roentgen; grain(s); gravity; gray (unit)
gr− Gram-negative (bacteria)
gr+ Gram-positive (bacteria)
grad gradient; graduate(d)
GRAE generally regarded as effective
gran *granulatus* (L) granulated
GRAS generally regarded as safe (with reference to food additives)
grav gravid (pregnant); gravity
grd ground
GRF growth hormone-releasing factor
GRID gay-related immunodeficiency
GRIF growth hormone release-inhibiting factor
gros *grossus* (L) coarse
GrP Gram-positive
grp group
GRPS glucose-Ringer-phosphate solution
GS gastric shield; general surgery; glomerular sclerosis
g/s gallons per second
GSA general somatic afferent (nerve)
GSBG gonadal steroid-binding globulin
GSC gravity settling culture (plate)
GSCN giant serotonin-containing neuron
GSD genetically significant dose (of X-rays); glycogen storage disease
GSE general somatic efferent (nerve); glutagen sensitive enteropathy
GSF galactosaemic fibroblasts
GSH glutathione (reduced form)
GSoA Gerontological Society of America
GSP galvanic skin potential
GSR galvanic skin response; generalized Shwartzman reaction
GSS gamete shedding substance
GSSG glutathione (oxidized form)
GSSG-R glutathione reductase
GST graphic stress telethermometry
GSW gunshot wound
GSWA gunshot wound to the abdomen
GT generation time; genetic therapy; glucose tolerance; glycityrosine; greater trochanter; group therapy
gt *gutta* (L) drop

g/t granulation time; granulation tissue
GT1 glycogenosis type 1
GTF glucose tolerance factor
GTH gonadotrophic hormone
GTN gestational trophoblastic neoplasia; glomerulo-tubulo-nephritis
GTO Golgi tendon organ
GTP glutamyl transpeptidase; guanosine triphosphate
GTR granulocyte turnover rate
GTT glucose tolerance test
gtt *guttae* (L) drops
GU gastric ulcer; genitourinary; glycogenic unit; gonococcal urethritis; gravitational ulcer
guid guidance
gutt *gutturi* (L) to the throat
gutt quibusd *guttis quibusdam* (L) with a few drops
guttat *guttatim* (L) drop by drop
GV gentian violet; gross virus nodules
GVA general visceral afferent (nerve)
GVBD germinal vesicle breakdown
GVE general visceral efferent (nerve)
GVG gamma-vinyl-GABA
GVH graft versus host (reaction)
GVHD graft versus host disease
GVHR graft versus host reaction
Gvty gingivectomy
GW germ warfare; glycerine in water
Gy gray (SI)
GYN gynaecologist(-ology)

H

H Hauch antigen; haemagglutination; heart or heart disease; heavy; henry (unit of electrical inductance) (SI); heroin; Holzknecht unit; homosexual; hormone; horse (in veterinary medicine); hospital; hour; human; hydrogen; hydrolysis; hygiene; hyoscine (scopolamine); hypermetropia; hypodermic; mustard gas
h *haustus* (L) a draught; hecto (prefix) (SI); height; henry (unit of electrical inductance); *hora* (L) hour; horizontal
H⁺ hydrogen ion

¹H protium (light hydrogen)
²H deuterium (heavy hydrogen)
H₃ procaine hydrochloride
³H tritium
HA haemadsorption (test); haemagglutination; haemagglutinating activity; haemolytic anaemia; headache; hearing aid; hepatitis associated (virus); Heyden antibiotic; Hospital Apprentice; hyaluronic acid
Ha absolute hypermetropia
HA1 haemadsorption (virus, type 1)
HAA haemolytic anaemia antigen; hearing aid amplifier; hepatitis associated antigen; Hospital Activity Analysis
H&A Ins Health and Accident Insurance
HAc acetic acid
HAChT high/affinity choline transport
HAD haemadsorption; hospital administration(-ator)
HAE hereditary angioedema
haem haemolysis (with reference to blood fragility test)
haemat haematocrit; haematology
haematol haematologist(-ology)
haemorrh haemorrhage
HAGG hyperimmune antivariola gamma globulin
HAI haemagglutination inhibition
HaLV hamster leukaemia virus
halluc hallucination
HAM hearing aid microphone
HAN hyperplastic alveolar nodules
HANDICP handicapped
HANES Health and Nutrition Examination Survey
H antigens antigens localized in flagella of motile bacteria
HAO Hospitals, Administrators, and Organizations
HAP Health Alliance Plan; hydrolysed animal protein; Handicapped Aid Program
HAS highest asymptomatic (dose); hypertensive arteriosclerotic
H&ASHD hypertension and arteriosclerotic heart disease
HASP Hospital Admission and Surveillance Program
HAsP Health Aspects of Pesticides
HATH Heterosexual Attitudes Toward Homosexuality (scale)
haust *haustus* (L) of a draught
HAV hepatitis A virus
HB bundle of His; Health Board; heart block; hepatitis B
Hb haemoglobin
HbA adult haemoglobin

HBAb hepatitis B antibody
HBAg hepatitis B antigen
HB$_c$Ag hepatitis B core antigen
HBB Hospital Blood Bank
HBD has been drinking
HBE His bundle electrogram
HBF hepatic blood flow
HbF fetal haemoglobin
HBGM home blood glucose monitoring
HBIg hepatitis B immunoglobulin
HBO hyperbaric oxygen (therapy)
HbO$_2$ oxyhaemoglobin
HBP high blood pressure
HbP primitive (fetal) haemoglobin
HbS sickle-cell haemoglobin
HBsAG hepatitis B surface antigen
HBSS Hank's balanced salt solution
HBT human breast tumour
HBV hepatitis B virus
HC handicapped; hippocampus; home care; Hospital Corps; house call; hydrocarbon; hydrocortisone
HCA heart cell aggregate; hepatocellular adenoma; Hospital Corporation of America
HCAP handicapped
HCC hepatitis contagiosa canis (virus); hepatocellular carcinoma
HCD heavy chain disease (protein); homologous canine distemper (antiserum)
HCG human chorionic gonadotrophin
HCH hexachlorocyclohexane (benzene hexachloride)
HcImp hydrocolloid impression (dentistry)
HCL hairy cell leukaemia; human cultured lymphoblastoid (cells)
HCl hydrochloric acid
HCLF high carbohydrate, low fibre (diet)
HCP handicapped
H&CP Hospital and Community Psychiatry
HCN hydrocyanic acid
HCO$_3$ bicarbonate ion
HCRE Homeopathic Council for Research and Education
H'crit haematocrit
HCS Hospital Car Service; human chorionic somatomammotrophin (HPL)
HCSD Health Care Studies Division

HCT heart-circulation training; human chorionic (placental) thyrotrophin

Hct haematocrit

HCVD hypertensive cardiovascular disease

HD haemodialysis; haemolysing dose; Hajna-Damon (broth); Hansen's disease (leprosy); hearing distance; heart disease; herniated disc; high density; hip disarticulation; Hodgkin's disease; Huntington's disease

hd *hora decubitis* (L) at bedtime

HDA Huntington's Disease Association; hydroxydopamine

HDC histidine decarboxylase

HDCS human diploid cell strain

HDCV human diploid cell rabies vaccine

HDD Higher Dental Diploma

HDF human diploid fibroblasts

HDFP Hypertension Detection and Follow-up Program

HDL high density lipoprotein

HDL-c high density lipoprotein-cell surface (receptor)

HDLW distance at which a watch is heard with left ear

HDMTX high dose methotrexate

HDN haemolytic disease of the newborn

hDNA deoxyribonucleic acid, histone

HDP hexose diphosphate

HDRF Heart Disease Research Foundation

HDRW distance at which a watch is heard with right ear

HDS Hospital Discharge Survey

HDU haemodialysis unit

HE Hearing Examiner; hepatic encephalopathy; hereditary elliptocytosis; human enteric; hypogonadotrophic eunuchoidism

H&E haematoxylin and eosin; haemorrhage and exudate; heredity and environment

He helium

HEAT human erythrocyte agglutination test

hebdom *hebdomada* (L) a week

HEC Health Education Council (Brit)

HED *Haut-Einheits-Dosis* (Ger) unit skin dose (of roentgen rays)

HEENT head, ears, eyes, nose, and throat

HEK human embryonic kidney (cells)

HEL hen's egg-white lysozyme; human embryonic lung (cells); human erythroleukaemia

HeLa Helen Lake (tumour cells)

HELF human embryonic lung fibroblasts

HELLP haemolysis, elevated liver enzymes, and low platelet (count)

HELP Health Education Library Program; Health Emergency Loan Program (Planned Parenthood); Health Evaluation and Learning Program; Henry's Emergency Lessons for People; Heroin Emergency Life Project; Hospital Equipment Loan Project

HEMA Health Education Media Association

HEMAT haematology

hemi hemiparalysis; hemiplegia

HEMPAS hereditary erythroblastic multinuclearity with positive acidified serum (test)

HEP high egg passage (strain of virus); high energy phosphate; human epithelial cells

HEPA high efficiency particulate air (filter)

HEPES hydroxyethylpiperazine ethanesulphonic acid

HEPM human embryonic palatal mesenchymal (cells)

herb recent *herbarium recentium* (L) of fresh herbs

hered heredity

hern hernia(ted)

HERS Health Evaluation and Referral Service; National Heart Education Research Society

HES hypereosinophilic syndrome

HESCA Health Sciences Communications Association

HESO Hospital Educational Services Officer

HET Health Education Telecommunications (HHS); heterozygous

HEV health and environment

HEW Health, Education and Welfare (Dept of) (*now* HHS)

HF haemorrhagic factor; Hageman factor (in blood plasma); hard filled (capsules); hay fever; heart failure; high fat (diet); high frequency; human fibroblasts

H/F HeLa/fibroblast (hybrid)

hf half

HFC hard filled capsules; high frequency current

HFD Hospital Field Director

HFDK human fetal diploid kidney (cells)

HFI hereditary fructose intolerance

HFIF human fibroblast interferon

HFJV high-frequency jet ventilation

HFP hypofibrinogenic plasma

HFPPV high frequency positive pressure ventilation

HFR high frequency of recombination

Hfr high frequency

HFRS   haemorrhagic fever with renal syndrome
HFST   hearing-for-speech test (Brit)
HFT   high frequency transduction
HG   herpes gestationis; human gonadotrophin; human growth factor
Hg   haemoglobin; *hydrargyrum* (L) mercury
hg   hectogram (SI)
hgb   haemoglobin
HGA   homogentisate
HGF   hyperglycaemic-glycogenolytic factor (glucagon)
Hg-F   fetal haemoglobin
HGG   human gamma globulin
HGH   human growth hormone
HGMCR   human genetic mutant cell repository
HGO   hepatic glucose output
HH   hard of hearing; Henderson and Haggard (inhaler); holistic health; Home Help
HHA   Home Health Agency; hypothalamic-hypophyseal-adrenal
HHb   reduced haemoglobin
HHD   hypertensive heart disease
HHHO   hypotonia-hypomentia-hypogonadism-obesity
H+Hm   compound hypermetropic astigmatism
HHS   Department of Health and Human Services
HHSSA   Home Health Services and Staffing Association
HHT   hereditary haemorrhagic telangiectasia
HI   haemagglutination inhibition; Health Insurance; hepatobiliary imaging; Hospital Insurance; hydriotic acid
Hi   histidine
HIA   heat infusion agar
HIAA   hydroxyindole-acetic acid
HIBAC   Health Insurance Benefits Advisory Council
HIC   Heart Information Center
HID   headache, insomnia, depression (syndrome)
HIFBS   heat-inactivated fetal bovine serum
HIFC   hog intrinsic factor concentrate
HIg   human immunoglobulin
HII   Health Industries Institute; Health Insurance Institute
HIMA   Health Industries Manufacturers Association
H inf   hypodermoclysis infusion
Hint   Hinton (flocculation test for syphilis)
HIO   hypoiodism; iodic acid
HIOMT   hydroxyindol-O-methyl transferase

HIP Health Insurance Plan; Hospital Insurance Program
HIPE Hospital In-patient Enquiry (Brit)
HIPO Hospital Indicator for Physicians Orders
HIS Health Information Service; Health Interview Survey (NIH); Hospital Informations Systems
His histidine
HIST Hospital In-service Training
Hist history
Histol histology
HIT haemagglutination inhibition test (for pregnancy)
HJ Howell-Jolly (bodies)
HJR hepatojugular reflex (reflux)
HK hexokinase; human kidney (cells)
H-K hands to knee
HL half-life (of radioactive element); histocompatibility locus; Hodgkin's lymphoma; Hygienic Laboratory (see USHL); hypertrichosis lanuginosa
H/L hydrophile/lipophile (number)
Hl latent hypermetropia, hyperopia
hl hectolitre (SI)
H&L heart and lungs
HLA histocompatibility locus antigen; histocompatibility locus A (system); homologous leucocytic antibodies; human leucocyte antigen (system); Human Life Amendment
HLALD horse liver alcohol dehydrogenase
HL-A-LD human lymphocyte-antigen—lymphocyte defined
HL-A-SD human lymphocyte-antigen—serologically defined
HLB hydrophile-lipophile balance (with reference to surfactants); hypotonic lysis buffer
HLC Human Lactation Center
HLD hypersensitivity lung disease
HLF heat-labile factor
HLH human luteinizing hormone
HLN hyperplastic liver nodules
HLP hyperlipoproteinaemia
HLR heart-lung resuscitation
HLS Health Learning Systems
HLV herpes-like virus
HM hand movements; hydatidiform mole; hyperimmune mice
Hm manifest hypermetropia
hm hectometre (SI)

HMAC Health Manpower Advisory Council
HMAS hyperimmune mice ascitic (fluid)
HMB homatropine methobromide
HMC heroin, morphine, cocaine
HMD hyaline membrane disease
HME Health Media Education; heat, massage, exercise
HMG human menopausal gonadotrophin
HML human milk lysosome
HMM heavy meromyosin
HMMA 4-hydroxy-3-methoxymandelic acid
HMO Health Maintenance Organization; heart minute output
HMP hexose monophosphate
HMR histocytic medullary reticulosis
H-mRNA H-chain messenger ribonucleic acid
HMS Health Mobilization Series
HMT human molar thyrotrophin
HMX heat-massage-exercise
HN Head Nurse; Home Nursing; Hospitalman (Navy); human nutrition
hn *hoc nocte* (L) tonight
HNA heparin neutralizing activity
HNC hypothalamic-neurohypophyseal complex
HNP herniated nucleus pulposus
hnRNA heterogenous nuclear ribonucleic acid
HNS head, neck, and shaft (of a bone); Home Nursing Supervisor
HNV has not voided
HO House Officer
H/O history of
HoaRhLG horse anti-rhesus lymphocyte globulin
HoaTTG horse anti-tetanus toxoid globulin
HOC human ovarian cancer
HOCM hypertrophic obstructive cardiomyopathy
hoc vesp *hoc vespere* (L) this evening, tonight
HOD hyperbaric oxygen drenching
HofF height of fundus
HoIg horse immunoglobulin
Hoff Hoffman (reflex)
Homeop homeopathy
Homo homosexual
Homolat homolateral
HOOD hereditary osteo-onchodysplasia
HOP high oxygen pressure
HOPE health-oriented physical education

hor horizontal
hor decu *hora decubitus* (L) at bedtime
hor interim *horis intermediis* (L) at the intermediate hours
hor som *hori somni* (L) at bedtime
hor un spatio *horae unius spatio* (L) at the end of one hour
HOS human osteosarcoma
HoS horse serum
Hosp hospital
Hosp Ins hospital insurance
HOST hypo-osmotic shock treatment
HOT human old tuberculin
HP handicapped person; high potency; high power; high pressure; highly purified; Hospital Participation; hot pack or pad; House Physician; hydrostatic pressure; hyperparathyroidism; hyperphoria; hypertension + proteinuria
H&P history and physical (examination)
Hp haptoglobin
HPA hypothalamic-pituitary-adrenocortical
HPBC hyperpolarizing bipolar cell
HPC hippocampal pyramidal cell
HPD high protein diet
H-PD Hough-Powell digitizer
HPF high-power field
HPG human pituitary gonadotrophin
HPI history of present illness
HPL human parotid lysozyme; human peripheral lymphocyte; human placental lactogen
HPLC high-performance liquid chromatography
HPN hypertension
HPP hereditary pyropoikilocytosis
hPP human pancreatic polypeptide
HPr human prolactin
HPS high protein supplement
HPT human placenta thyrotrophin
HPV hypoxic pulmonary vasoconstriction
HPV-DE high-passage virus – duck embryo
HPV-DK high passage virus – dog kidney
HR haemorrhagic retinopathy; heart rate; heterosexual relations (scale); higher rate; Hospital Recruit
hr hour
HRA Health Resources Administration; heart rate audiometry

HRC horse red cells
HRE high resolution electrocardiography
HRG Health Research Group
HRIg human rabies immune globulin
HRL head rotated left
hRNA heterogeneous ribonucleic acid
HRP horseradish peroxidase
HRR head rotated right
HRRC Walt Disney Hearing Rehabilitation Research Center
HRS hormone receptor site
HRV human rotavirus
HS half strength; Hartmann's solution; head sling; heart sounds; Henoch-Schönlein (syndrome); hereditary spherocytosis; herpes simplex; homologous serum; horse serum; Hospital Ship; Hospital Staff; hour of sleep; House Supervisor; House Surgeon
hs *hora somni* (L) at bedtime
H&S hysterotomy and sterilization
HSA Health Services Administration; Health Systems Agency; horse serum albumin; Hospital Savings Association; human serum albumin
HSAA Health Sciences Advancement Award
HSAG HEPES-saline-albumin-gelatin
HSAS hypertrophic subaortic stenosis
HSC Health and Safety Commission (Brit)
HS-CoA coenzyme A (reduced)
HSD hydroxysteroid dehydrogenase
HSE Health and Safety Executive; herpes simplex encephalitis
HSF hypothalamic secretory factor
HSG herpes simplex genitalis; hysterosalpingogram
hSGF human skeletal growth factor
HSHP High School for Health Professions
HSJ Hôpital St Joseph (Paris)
HSL herpes simplex labialis
HSMHA Health Services and Mental Health Administration (HHS)
HSN hereditary sensory neuropathy
HSP Health Systems Plan (HHS); Hospital Service Plan (Brit); human serum prealbumin
HSQB Health Standards and Quality Bureau (HHS)
HSR homogeneous staining region
HSRC Human-Subjects Review Committee
HSRD hypertension secondary to renal disease

HSRI Health Systems Research Institute
HSS high speed supernatant; Hospital and Specialist Service; hypertrophic subaortic stenosis
HSTF human serum thymus factor
HSV herpes simplex virus
HSVE herpes simplex virus encephalitis
H&T hospitalization and treatment
HT *haustus* (L) a draught; heart; heart transplant; high temperature; home treatment; hospital train; Huhner test; human thrombin; hydrotherapy; hydroxytryptamine (serotonin); hypermetropia (with L or R); hypodermic tablet; hypothalamus
ht heart tones; height; high tension
HTA hypophysiotropic area (of the hypothalamus)
HTACS human thyroid adenyl-cyclase stimulator
HTB hot tub bath
HTC hepatoma cells; homozygous typing cells
HTD human therapeutic dose
HTF heterothyrotrophic factors
HTH homoeostatic thymus hormone
HTLA high-titre, low acidity
HTLV human T-cell leukaemia virus
HTN hypertension(-sive)
HTO hospital transfer order
HTS human thyroid stimulator
HTSH human thyroid stimulating hormone
HTST high temperature – short time (pasteurization)
HTV herpes type virus
HU haemagglutinating unit; haemolytic unit; Harvard University; hyperaemia unit
HUC hypouricaemia
HUS haemolytic uraemic syndrome
HV herpesvirus; hyperventilation
HVA homovanillic acid
HVC Health Visitor's Certificate (Brit)
HVc hyperstriatum ventrale, pars caudale
HVD hypertensive vascular disease
HVG host versus graft (response)
HVH herpesvirus hominis
HVJ haemagglutinating virus of Japan
HVL half value layer
HVR hypoxic ventilatory response
HVS herpesvirus of Saimiri
HW housewife
HWC Health and Welfare, Canada

HWS hot water soluble
HWY hundred woman years (of exposure)
Hx history; hypoxanthine
Hy hypermetropia; hypothenar
HYD hydrated; hydroxyurea
hydr hydraulic
hydrarg *hydrargyrum* (L) mercury
Hydro hydrotherapy
Hyg hygiene
Hygst Hygienist
HYL hydroxylysine
HYP hypnosis
Hyp hydroxyproline; hyperresonance; hypertrophy
Hypn hypertension
hypno hypnosis, hypnotism
Hypo hypodermic injection
Hypox hypophysectomized
Hypro hydroxyproline
hys hysteria(-ical)
Hz hertz

I

I incisor (permanent); index; indicated; induction; inhibitor; intensity of magnetism; internist; iodine
i incisor (deciduous); insoluble; optically inactive
^{125}**I**, ^{130}**I**, ^{131}**I** radioactive iodine
IA immune adherence; impedance angle; indolaminergic-accumulating (cells); indulin agar; infected area; inferior angle; intra-arterial; intra-articular; intra-atrial; intra-auricular
Ia immune region associated antigen
IAA indole-3-acetic acid; International Antituberculosis Association
IAB Industrial Accident Board; intra-abdominal; intra-aorta balloon
IABC intra-aorta balloon counterpulsation
IABP intra-aorta balloon pump
IAC intra-arterial chemotherapy
IACS International Academy of Cosmetic Surgery
IACVF International Association of Cancer Victims and Friends

IAD   internal absorbed dose

IADR   International Association for Dental Research

IAEA   International Atomic Energy Agency

IAFI   infantile amaurotic familial idiocy

IAG   International Association of Gerontology

IAGP   International Association of Geographic Pathology

IAGUS   International Association of Genito-Urinary Surgeons

IAH   implantable artificial heart

IAHA   immune adherence haemoagglutination

IAHP   International Association of Heart Patients

IAHS   International Association for Hospital Security

IAL   International Association of Laryngectomees

IAM   Institute of Aviation Medicine

IAMM   International Association of Medical Museums

IAO   immediately after onset; intermittent aortic occlusion

IAP   Institute of Animal Physiology (Brit); International Academy of Pathology; International Academy of Proctology

IAPB   International Association for Prevention of Blindness

IAPM   International Academy of Preventative Medicine

IAPP   International Association for Preventative Pediatrics

AIRC   International Agency for Research on Cancer

IAS   intra-amniotic saline (infusion)

IASD   interatrial septal defect

IASHS   Institute for Advanced Study in Human Sexuality

IASL   International Association for Study of the Liver

IASP   International Association for the Study of Pain

IAT   iodine azide test

IAV   intra-arterial vasopressin

IB   immune body; inclusion body; index of body build; infectious bronchitis; Institute of Biology (Brit)

ib   *ibidem* (L) in the same place

IBA   Industrial Biotechnology Association

IBC   Institutional Biosafety Committee; iodine-binding capacity

IBD   inflammatory bowel disease

IBE   International Bureau for Epilepsy

IBED   InterAfrican Bureau for Epizootic Diseases

iB-EP   immunoreactive beta-endomorphin

IBF   immature brown fat (cells)

IBI intermittent bladder irrigation

ibid *ibidem* (L) in the same place

IBK infectious bovine keratoconjunctivitis

IBMP International Board of Medicine and Psychology

IBP International Biological Program; iron-binding protein

IBPMS indirect blood pressure measuring system

IBR infectious bovine rhinotracheitis

IBRO International Brain Research Organization

IBRV infective bovine rhinotracheitis virus

IBS irritable bowel syndrome

IBT Industrial Bio-Test Laboratories

IBV infectious bronchitis vaccine

IBW ideal body weight

IC immune complex; inferior colliculus; inorganic carbon; inspiratory capacity; inspiratory centre; intensive care; intercostal; interstitial cells; intracardiac; intracellular; intracerebral; intracutaneous (injection); islet cells (of the pancreas); Institutional Care (Brit)

ic *inter cibos* (L) between meals

ICA Institute of Clinical Analysis; islet cell antibodies

ICAA International Council on Alcohol and Addictions; Invalid Children's Aid Association

ICAMI International Committee Against Mental Illness

ICAV intracavity

ICBP intracellular binding proteins

ICC immunocytochemistry; Information Centre Complex; Internal Conversion Coefficient (radiology)

ICCM idiopathic congestive cardiomyopathy

ICCR International Committee for Contraceptive Research

ICCU Intermediate Coronary Care Unit

ICD immune complex disease; Institute for Crippled and Disabled; International Center for the Disabled; International Classification of Diseases; International College of Dentists; intrauterine contraceptive device

ICDA International Classification of Diseases, Adapted

ICDH isocitric dehydrogenase

ICEA International Childbirth Education Association

ICF indirect centrifugal flotation; Intensive Care Facility; Intermediate Care Facility; International Cardiology Foundation; intracellular fluid; intravascular coagulation and fibrinolysis (syndrome)

ICF(M)A International Cystic Fibrosis (Mucoviscidosis) Association

ICFMR Intermediate Care Facility for the Mentally Retarded

ICG indocyanine green

ICH infectious canine hepatitis

ICLA International Committee on Laboratory Animals

ICM inner cell mass; intercostal margin; International Confederation of Midwives

ICN Intensive Care Nursery; International Council of Nurses

ICP Infection-control Practitioner; intracranial pressure

ICPA International Commission for the Prevention of Alcoholism

ICPI Intersociety Committee on Pathology Information

I, C, PM, M incisors, canines, premolars, molars (When each is followed by a fraction, the entire expression is the formula of permanent dentition)

ICR distance between iliac crests; Institute for Cancer Research; International Congress of Radiology; intracranial reinforcement

ICRC International Committee of the Red Cross

ICRD Index of Codes for Research Drugs

ICRETT International Cancer Research Technology Transfer

ICREW International Cancer Research Workshop

ICRF Imperial Cancer Research Fund (Brit)

ICRFSDD Independent Citizens Research Foundation for the Study of Degenerative Diseases

ICRP International Commission on Radiological Protection

ICRU International Commission on Radiation Units and Measurements

ICS Imperial College of Science (Brit); impulse-conducting system; Intensive Care, Surgical; intercostal space; International Cardiovascular Study; International College of Surgeons; International Craniopathic Society; intracranial stimulation

ICSH International Committee for Standardization in Haematology; interstitial cell-stimulating hormone (LH)

ICSS intracranial self-stimulation

ICSU International Council of Scientific Unions

ICT icterus; indirect Coombs's test; inflammation of connective tissue; insulin coma therapy

iCT immunoreactive calcitonin

ICTH International Committee on Thrombosis and

Homeostasis
ICTMM International Congress on Tropical Medicine and Malaria
ICTV International Committee on Taxonomy of Viruses
ICU Intensive Care Unit
ICV intracerebroventricular
ICVS International Cardiovascular Society
ID immunodeficiency; immunodiffusion; inclusion disease; index of discrimination; individual dose; infectious disease(s); infective dose; inhibitory dose; injected dose; inside diameter; intradermal(ly)
id *idem* (L) the same
ID$_{50}$ median infective dose
I&D incision and drainage
id ac *idem ac* (L) the same as
IDAMIS Integrated Dose Abuse Management Informational Systems
IDARP Integrated Drug Abuse Reporting Process
IDDM insulin-dependent diabetes mellitus
IDIC Internal Dose Information Center
IDK internal derangement of knee (joint)
IDL intermediate density lipoprotein
IDM indirect method
idon vehic *idoneo vehiculo* (L) in a suitable vehicle
IDP immunodiffusion procedures; inosine diphosphate
IDPH idiopathic pulmonary haemosiderosis
IDPN iminodiproprionitrile
IDS Investigative Dermatological Society
IDSA Infectious Disease Society of America
IDT International Diagnostic Technology
IDU iododeoxyuridine (idoxuridine)
IdUA iduronic acid
IDV intermittent demand ventilation
IE *Immunitäts Einheit* (Ger) *immunizing* unit; immunoelectrophoresis; intake energy (unit of food)
ie *id est* (L) that is
IEA immunoelectroadsorption; International Epidemiological Association; intravascular erythrocyte aggregation
IEC injection electrode catheter; intra-epithelial carcinoma; ion exchange chromatography
IEE inner enamel epithelium
IEF International Eye Foundation
IEL intraepithelial lymphocytes
IEM inborn error of metabolism

IEP immunoelectrophoresis; isoelectric point
IF immunofluorescence (test); infrared; inhibiting factor; interferon; intermediate frequency; interstitial fluid; intrinsic factor
IFA immunofluorescence assay; indirect fluorescent antibody; International Fertility Association; International Filariasis Association
IFCR International Foundation for Cancer Research
IFCS inactivated fetal calf serum
IFFH International Foundation for Family Health
IFGO International Federation of Gynecology and Obstetrics
IFHP International Federation of Health Professionals
IFHPMSM International Foundation for Hygiene, Preventative Medicine, and Social Medicine
IFLrA recombinant human leucocyte interferon A
IFM intrafusal muscle
IFMBE International Federation for Medical and Biological Engineering
IFME International Federation for Medical Electronics
IFMP International Federation for Medical Psychotherapy
IFPM International Federation of Physical Medicine
IFMSA International Federation of Medical Student Associations
IFMSS International Federation of Multiple Sclerosis Societies
IFN interferon
If nec if necessary
IFR infrared
IFRP International Fertility Research Program
IFSM International Federation of Sports Medicine
IFT International Frequency Tables
Ig immunoglobulin, γ-globulin
IgA immunoglobulin A
IgD immunoglobulin D
IgE immunoglobulin E
IGF insulin-like growth factor
IgG immunoglobulin G
IGH immunoreactive growth hormone
IgM immunoglobulin M
IGS inappropriate gonadotrophin secretion
IH immediate hypersensitivity; Industrial Hygienist; infectious hepatitis; inhibiting hormone; In-patient Hospital; iron haematoxylin

toneal(ly); ionization potential; iso-electric point

IPA Individual Practice Association; International Pediatric Association; International Psychoanalytical Association

I-para primipara

IPC International Poliomyelitis Congress

IPCS intrauterine progesterone contraceptive system (an IUD)

IPD intermittent peritoneal dialysis; Inventory of Psychosocial Development

IPEH intravascular papillary endothelial hyperplasia

iPGE immunoreactive prostaglandin E

IPH interphalangeal

IPM impulses per minute; inches per minute

IPP L'Institut Pasteur Productions

IPPA inspection, palpation, percussion, auscultation

IPPB intermittent positive pressure breathing

IPPB/I intermittent positive pressure breathing/inspiratory

IPPF International Planned Parenthood Federation

IPPNW International Physicians for the Prevention of Nuclear War

IPPR intermittent positive pressure respiration

IPPV intermittent positive pressure ventilation

IPQ intimacy potential quotient

IPS intraperitoneal shock

ips inches per second

IPSP inhibitory post synaptic potential

IPTH immunoreactive parathyroid hormone

IPU Inpatient Unit

IPV inactivated poliomyelitis vaccine; infectious pustular vaginitis; infectious pustular vulvovaginitis (of cattle)

IQ intelligence quotient

IQ&S iron, quinine, and strychnine

IR immune response; immunization rate; immunoreactive; inferior rectus (muscle); infrared; insoluble residue; internal resistance

I-R Ito-Reenstierna (reaction)

Ir iridium

IRA immunoregulatory alpha-globulin

IRC International Red Cross

IRCC International Red Cross Committee

IRDS idiopathic respiratory distress syndrome

IRGH immunoreactive growth hormone

IRGI immunoreactive glucagon

IRH Institute for Research in Hypnosis; Institute of Religion and Health
IRI immunoreactive insulin
IRICU Intermountain Respiratory Intensive Care Unit
IRIg insulin reactive immunoglobulin
IRIS International Research Information Service
IRM innate releasing mechanism; Institute of Rehabilitation Medicine
IRMA immunoradiometric assay
IRMP Intermountain Regional Medical Program
iRNA immune ribonucleic acid
IRO International Refugee Organization
IROS ipsilateral routing of signal
IRP immunoreactive proinsulin; International Reference Preparation
IRR irritant(-ation)
IRRD Institute for Research in Rheumatic Diseases
IRRG irrigated(-tion)
IRS International Rhinologic Society
IRU Industrial Rehabilitation Unit; interferon reference unit
IRV inspiratory reserve volume
IS immune serum; immunosuppressive; intercostal space; intraspinal; invalided from service
is island
I-10-S invert sugar (10%) in saline
ISA Instrument Society of America; iodinated serum albumin
ISADH inappropriate secretion of antidiuretic hormone
ISBI International Society for Burn Injuries
ISBP International Society for Biochemical Pharmacology
ISBT International Society for Blood Transfusion
ISC insoluble collagen; International Society of Cardiology; International Society of Chemotherapy; International Statistical Classification; interstitial cells
ISCM International Society of Cybernetic Medicine
ISCP International Society of Clinical Pathology
ISD Information Services Division (Scottish Health Service); inhibited sexual desire
ISE inhibited sexual excitement; International Society of Endocrinology; International Society of Endoscopy
ISEK International Society of Electromyographic Kinesiology
ISF interstitial fluid

ISG immune serum globulin
ISGE International Society of Gastroenterology
ISH International Society of Hematology
ISI infarct size index; injury severity index; Institute for Scientific Information; International Sensitivity Index; interstimulus interval
ISKDC International Society of Kidney Diseases in Children
ISM International Society of Microbiologists; intersegmental muscles
ISMED International Society on Metabolic Eye Disorders
ISMH International Society of Medical Hydrology
ISMHC International Society of Medical Hydrology and Climatology
ISN International Society of Nephrology; International Society of Neurochemistry
ISO International Standards Organization
Is of Lang islands of Langerhans
isol isolate(-tion)
isom isometric
ISP distance between iliac spines; intraspinal
ISPO International Society for Prosthetics and Orthotics
ISPT interspecies ovum penetration test
isq *in status quo* (L) unchanged
ISR Information Storage and Retrieval; Institute for Sex Research; Institute of Surgical Research (Army)
ISRM International Society of Reproductive Medicine
ISS International Society of Surgery
IST insulin shock therapy; International Society on Toxicology
ISTD International Society of Tropical Dermatology
ISU International Society of Urology
I-sub inhibitor substance
ISY intrasynovial
IT immunity test; inhalation therapy; intrathoracic; ischial tuberosity
I/T intensity/duration
ITA International Tuberculosis Association
ITC Interagency Testing Committee
ITc International Table calorie
ITE in the ear (hearing aid)
ITh intrathecal (intraspinal) (with reference to injections)
ITLC instant thin-layer chromatography

ITP idiopathic thrombocytopenic purpura; inosine triphosphate

ITR intraocular tension recorder; intratracheal

ITT insulin tolerance test

IU immunizing unit; international unit; intrauterine; in utero

IUB International Union of Biochemistry

IUBS International Union of Biological Sciences

IUC idiopathic ulcerative colitis

IUCD intrauterine contraceptive device

IUD intrauterine death; intrauterine device

IUFB intrauterine foreign body

IUGR intrauterine growth retardation

IUP intrauterine pressure

IUPAC International Union of Pure and Applied Chemistry

IUPHAR International Union of Pharmacology

IUPS International Union of Physiological Sciences

IURES International Union of Reticuloendothelial Societies

IUT intrauterine transfusion

IUTM International Union Against Tuberculosis (*Mycobacterium*)

IUVDT International Union against Venereal Diseases and the Treponematoses

IV interventricular; intervertebral; intravenous(ly); intraventricular

iv iodine value

IVBAT intravascular bronchioalveolar tumour

IVC individually viable cells; inferior vena cava; intravenous cholangiogram

IVCD intraventricular conduction defect

IVD intervertebral disc

IVF intravascular fluid

IVGTT intravenous glucose tolerance test

IVH intravenous hyperalimentation; intraventricular haemorrhage

IVJC intervertebral joint complex

IVN intravenous nutrition

IVP intravenous push; intravenous pyelogram

IVPB intravenous piggyback

IVPD *in vitro* protein digestibility

IVR internal visual reference; isolated volume responders

IVRD *in vitro* rumen digestibility

IVS   interventricular septum
IVSA   International Veterinary Students Association
IVSD   interventricular septal defect
IVT   intravenous transfusion; intraventricular
IVV   intravenous vasopressin
I-5-W invert sugar (5%) in water
IYDP   International Year of Disabled Persons
IYS   inverted Y-suspensor
IZS   insulin zinc suspension

J

J   Jewish; joint; joule (SI); journal; juice; juvenile
j   In prescription writing, used as a Roman numeral as the
           equivalent of 'i' for *one, or* at the end of a number (e.g.
           j, ij, iij, vij)
JA   juxta-articular
JAI   juvenile amaurotic idiocy
JAMA   Journal of the American Medical Association
jaund jaundice
JBE   Japanese B encephalitis
JCAE   Joint Committee on Atomic Energy (US)
JCAH   Joint Commission on Accreditation of Hospitals
JCAST Joint Committee on Archives of Science and
           Technology
JCC   Joint Committee on Contraception
jct   junction
JD   juvenile diabetes
JDC   Joslin Diabetes Center
JDF   Juvenile Diabetes Foundation
JDM   juvenile diabetes mellitus
JE   Japanese encephalitis
JEE   Japanese equine encephalitis
jej   jejunum
JEN   Journal of Emergency Nursing
jentac *jentaculum* (L) breakfast
JER   Japanese erection ring
JG   juxtaglomerular
JGA   juxtaglomerular apparatus
JH   juvenile hormone (of insects)
JHM   J Howard Mueller virus
JHMO   Junior Hospital Medical Officer

JHU Johns Hopkins University
JJ jaw jerk
JMH John Milton Hagen (antibody)
JMSB John Milton Society for the Blind
JNA Jena Nomina Anatomica (*see* INA)
JND just noticeable difference
jnt joint
JOD juvenile onset diabetes
Jour journal
JPSA Joint Program for the Study of Abortions
JRA juvenile rheumatoid arthritis
JRC Junior Red Cross
JrNAD Junior National Association for the Deaf
JS Junkman-Schoeller (unit of thyrotrophin)
jt joint
jucund *jucunde* (L) pleasantly
juv juvenile
JV jugular vein
JVP jugular vein pulse
JUXT *juxta* (L) near

K

K absolute zero; electrostatic capacity; capsular antigen (from Kapsel); ionization constant; *kalium* (L) potassium; kallikrein inhibiting unit; kanamycin; Kelvin (temperature scale); kelvin (SI unit of temperature)
k constant; kilo (prefix) (SI); kilogram
ϰ kappa
K-10 gastric tube
17-K 17-ketosteroids
KA alkaline phosphatase; ketoacidosis; King-Armstrong (units)
K/A ketogenic to antiketogenic ratio
ka kathode (cathode)
KAAD mixture kerosene, alcohol, acetic acid, dioxane mixture
Kal *kalium* (L) potassium
KAP knowledge, aptitude and practices (with reference to fertility)
kat katal (enzyme unit)
KAU King-Armstrong unit

KB ketone bodies; knee brace
kb kilobase
KC kathodal (cathodal) closing
kc kilocycle
Kcal kilocalorie (1000 calories, or 1 Calorie)
KCC kathodal (cathodal) closing contraction
kCi kilocurie
kcps kilocycles per second
kc/s kilocycles per second
KCT kathodal (cathodal) closing tetanus
KD kathodal (cathodal) duration; Kawasaki disease; killed
KDSM keratizing desquamative squamous metaplasia
KDT kathodal (cathodal) duration tetanus
KE Kendall's compound E (cortisone); kinetic energy
K$_e$ exchangeable body potassium
keV kiloelectron-volt
KF Kenner-faecal medium
kf Symbol indicating flocculation speed in antigen-antibody reactions
KFD Kyasanur Forest disease (of South India)
kg kilogram (SI)
kg-cal kilocalorie (large calorie) (see Kcal)
KG-1 Koeffler Golde-1 (cell line)
kg-m kilogram-metre
kgps kilogram per second
KGS ketogenic steroid
KHB Krebs-Henseleit bicarbonate buffer
KHb potassium haemoglobinate
KHF Korean haemorrhagic fever
KHP Honorary Physician to the King (Brit)
KHS Honorary Surgeon to the King (Brit)
kHz kilohertz
KI Krönig's isthmus; potassium iodide
KIA Kligler iron agar (medium)
KIC ketoisocaproate
kilo kilogram; kilometre
KIMSV Kirsten murine sarcoma virus
KIU kallikrein inactivation unit
KJ knee jerk
KK knee kick (knee jerk)
KL kidney lobe
kl kilolitre (SI)
KL bac Klebs-Löffler bacillus (diphtheria bacillus)
Klebs *Klebsiella*

KLH keyhole limpet haemocyanin
KLS kidney, liver, spleen
km kilometre (SI)
kMc kilomegacycle
K-MCM potassium-containing minimal capacitation medium
KMEF keratin, myosin, epidermin, fibrin (class of proteins)
kmps kilometres per sec
KNL Darrow's solution (for anti-diarrhoea potassium therapy)
KO knocked out
KOM Kentucky, Ohio, Michigan (Medical Library Network)
KP Kaufmann-Peterson base; keratitis precipitates; keratitis punctata
K-P Kaiser-Permanente (diet)
KPI karyopyknotic index
KR Kopper Reppart (medium)
Kr krypton
KRP Kolmer test with Reiter protein
KS Kaposi's sarcoma; ketosteroid
KSCN potassium thiocyanate (broth)
KStJ Knight Commander, Order of St John of Jerusalem
K stoff chloromethyl chloroformate
KTSA Kahn Test of Symbol Arrangement
KUB kidney and upper bladder; kidney, ureter and bladder
kV kilovolt (SI)
kVA kilovolt-ampere (SI)
KVBA kanamycin-vancomycin blood agar
kVcp kilovolt constant potential
KVLBA kanamycin-vancomycin laked blood agar
kVp kilovolts peak
kW kilowatt (SI)
kW-hr kilowatt-hour

L

L Avogadro's constant; coefficient of induction; *Lactobacillus;* lambert (unit of luminance); Latin; left; lethal; lewisite; *liber* (L) book; *libra* (L) pound   licensed to practise; light; light (chain of protein molecules); light sense; lilac; lime; limen (threshold); lingual; low (when followed by another abbr., e.g. LBP); lower, lowest; Heat labile component of protein antigen of vaccinia and variola viruses

l laevorotatory; left eye; length; lethal; litre (SI); long; longitudinal (with reference to sections); lumen

λ lambda

L- laevorotatory; A chemical prefix (small capital) which designates that a substance has the configuration of L-glyceraldehyde; In carbohydrate nomenclature, the symbol designates the configuration family of the *highest numbered* asymmetric carbon atom, as in L-rhamnose; In amino acid nomenclature, the symbol designates the configuration family of the *lowest numbered* asymmetric carbon atom, as in L-threonine

L_1, L_2 first lumbar vertebra, second lumbar vertebra, etc

L/3 lower third (with reference to long bones)

L_+ limes death; *limes tod*

L_0 limes zero; *limes nul*

l Chemical abbreviation for *laevo*, to the left or counter-clockwise, especially with reference to direction in which a plane of polarized light is rotated

LA latex agglutination; left angle (angulation) (orthopaedics); left atrium; left auricle; leucine aminopeptidase; leucoagglutinating; linguo-axial; local anaesthesia; long-acting (with reference to drugs); low alcohol

L&A light and accommodation (with reference to reaction of pupils)

La labial

la *lege artis* (L) according to the art

LAAM l-acetyl-α-methadol (levomethadyl acetate)

LAAO L-amino acid oxidase

lab laboratory; rennet (Ger)

lab proc laboratory procedure

LABS Laboratory Admission Baseline Studies

LAC La Crosse subtype encephalitis; linguo-axiocervical

LaC labiocervical

lac laceration(s)

LAD lactic acid dehydrogenase; left axis deviation; lipoamide dehydrogenase

LADA left-acromio-dorso-anterior (position of fetus)

LADP left-acromio-dorso-posterior (position of fetus)

LAE left atrial enlargement

laev *laevus* (L) left

LAF laminar air flow
LAG linguo-axiogingival; lymphangiography
LaG labiogingival
lag *lagena* (L) flask, bottle
LAH left anterior hemiblock; left atrial hypertrophy; Licentiate of Apothecaries Hall, Dublin
LaI labioincisal
LAIT latex agglutination inhibition test (for pregnancy)
LaL labiolingual
LAM lymphangioleiomyomatosis
lam laminectomy
LAO Licentiate of the Art of Obstetrics
LAP leucine aminopeptidase; leucocyte alkaline phosphatase; lyophilized anterior pituitary
lap laparotomy
lapid *lapideum* (L) stony
LAR laryngology
lar left arm reclining or recumbent
LARC leucocyte automatic recognition computer
Laryngol laryngologist(-ology)
LAS Laboratory Automation System; linear alkylate sulphonate; local adaptation syndrome
LASER light amplification by stimulated emission of radiation
L-ASP L-asparaginase
LAT latex agglutination test
lat lateral
lat admov *lateri admoveatum* (L) let it be applied to the side
LATCH Literature Attached to Charts (Nursing Program)
lat dol *lateri dolenti* (L) to the painful side
LATS long-acting thyroid stimulator
LATS-P long-acting thyroid stimulator-protector
LB leiomyoblastoma; low back (disorder)
L&B left and below
lb *libra* (L) pound
LBBsB left bundle branch system block
LBCD left border cardiac dullness
LBCF Laboratory Branch Complement Fixation (test)
LBD left border of dullness (of heart to percussion)
LBF *Lactobacillus bulgaricus* factor (pantetheine); liver blood flow
LBH length, breadth, height
LBL lymphoblastic lymphoma

LBM   lean body mass
LBP   low back pain; low blood pressure
LBS   lactobacillus selector (agar)
LBW   low birth weight
LC   Langerhan's cells; life care; linguocervical
LCA   left coronary artery
LCAR   late cutaneous anaphylactic reaction
LCAT   lecithin-cholesterol acyltransferase
LCC   lactose coliform count
LCCS   low cervical Caesarean section
LCFA   long-chain fatty acid
LCGU   local cerebral glucose utilization
LCh   Licentiate in Surgery
LCL   Levinthal-Coles-Lillie (bodies)
LCM   left costal margin; lowest common multiple; lymphocytic choriomeningitis
LCME   Liaison Committee on Medical Education
LCMV   lymphocytic choriomeningitis virus
LCP   long-chain polysaturated (fatty acids)
LCPS   Licentiate of the College of Physicians and Surgeons
LCS   Life Care Services
LCT   lymphocytotoxicity test
LCx   left circumflex coronary artery
LD   lactate dehydrogenase; legionnaire's disease; lethal dose; light-dark; light difference, perception of; linguodistal; living donor; Lombard-Dowell broth medium; long day (in plant growth); low density; lymphocytically determined
LD$_{50}$ median lethal dose
LDA   left dorso-anterior (position of fetus)
LDB   legionnaires' disease bacterium
LD-EYA   Lombard-Dowell egg yolk agar
LD-NEYA   Lombard-Dowell neomycin egg yolk agar
LDH   lactate dehydrogenase
LDL   low-density lipoprotein
LDP   left dorsoposterior (position of fetus)
LDS   Licentiate in Dental Surgery
LDSc   Licentiate in Dental Science
LDUB   long double upright brace
LE   left eye; lower extremity; lupus erythematosus
Le   Leonard (unit for cathode rays)
Lect   lecturer
leg   legal(ly)
leg com   legally committed

LEL lowest effect level (of toxicity)
LEM lateral eye movements; Leibovitz-Emory (medium); leucocyte endogenous mediator
lenit *leniter* (L) gently
LEP low egg passage (strain of virus); lipoprotein electrophoresis
Lept *Leptospira*
LES Lawrence Experiment Station (agar); local excitatory state; Locke egg serum (medium); lower esophageal sphincter
LET lineal energy transfer
Leu leucine
LEV Leibovitz-Emory medium (for viral cultures)
lev *levis* (L) light
l/ext lower extremity
Lf limit of flocculation
lf low frequency
LFA left frontoanterior (left mentoanterior) (position of fetus)
LFD least fatal dose (of a toxin); low-fat diet
LFH left femoral hernia
LFP left frontoposterior (left mentoposterior) (position of fetus)
LFPS Licentiate of the Faculty of Physicians and Surgeons
LFT latex fixation test; left frontotransverse (left mentotransverse) (position of fetus); liver function test; low frequency transduction
LFV Lassa-fever virus
LG linguogingival
lg large
LGA large for gestational age
LGd dorsal lateral geniculate (nucleus)
LGH lactogenic hormone
LGI large glucagon immunoreactivity
LGL large granular leucocytes; Lown-Ganong-Levine syndrome
LGT Langat encephalitis; late generalized tuberculosis
LGV lymphogranuloma venereum
LH left hand; left hyperphoria; lower half; lues hereditaria; luteinizing hormone (ICSH)
LHC left hypochondrium; Local Health Councils (Scotland)
LHI lipid hydrocarbon inclusions
LHM lysuride hydrogen maleate

LHMP Life Health Monitoring Program
LHR leucocyte histamine release (test)
l-hr lumen hour
LHRF luteinizing hormone-releasing factor
LHS left hand side; left heart strain
LHT left hypertropia
LI linguoincisal
LI, LII, LIII (see lues)
Li lithium
LIA leukaemia cell-derived inhibitory activity; lysine iron agar
lib *libra* (L) pound
LIBC latent iron-binding capacity
LIC limiting isorrhoeic concentration
Lic Licentiate
LICM left intercostal margin
LicMed Licentiate in Medicine
LIF left iliac fossa; leucocytosis-inducing factor
lig ligament
LIH left inguinal hernia
lim limit
lin linear
LINES long interspersed repeated segments (of DNA)
linim liniment
LINK Literature in Nursing Kardex
Linn Linnaeus, Linnaean
Lip lipoate (lipoic acid)
liq *liquor* (L) a liquor or liquid
LIRBM liver, iron, red bone marrow
LIS lobular in situ (carcinoma)
lit literal(ly)
LIV liver battery test (dentistry); living
LKQCPI Licentiate of the King and Queen's College of Physicians in Ireland
LKS liver, kidney, spleen
LKV laked kanamycin vancomycin (agar)
LL left lower; lower leg; lower lid
LLBCD left lower border of cardiac dullness
LLD *Lactobacillus lactis* Dorner factor (vitamin B_{12})
LLE left lower extremity
LLF Laki-Lorand factor (fibrinase); left lateral femoral (site of injection)
LLL left lower eyelid; left lower lobe (of lung)
LLM localized leucocyte mobilization
LLO legionella-like organism(s)

LLQ left lower quadrant (of abdomen)
LLR left lateral rectus eye muscle
LM laryngeal muscle; lateral malleolus; legal medicine; Licentiate in Medicine; Licentiate in Midwifery; light minimum; linguomesial; lipid mobilizing (hormone); longitudinal muscle; lower motor (neuron)
lm lumen
LMA left mentoanterior (position of fetus)
LMB leiomyoblastoma
LMBBS Lawrence-Moon-Biedl-Bardet syndrome
LMC lymphomyeloid complex
LMCAD left main coronary artery disease
LMCC Licentiate of the Medical Council of Canada
LMD local medical doctor
LMed&Ch Licentiate in Medicine and Surgery
LML large and medium lymphocytes; left mediolateral (with reference to episiotomy)
LMM light meromyosin; *Lactobacillus* maintenance medium
LMN lower motor neuron
LMNL lower motor neuron lesion
LMP last menstrual period; left mentoposterior (position of fetus); lumbar puncture
LMR left medial rectus (eye muscle)
LMRCP Licentiate in Midwifery of the Royal College of Physicians
LMS leiomyosarcoma; Licentiate in Medicine and Surgery
LMSSA Licentiate in Medicine and Surgery of the Society of Apothecaries, London
LMT left mentotransverse (position of fetus)
In logarithm, natural
LNI log neutralization index
LNMP last normal menstrual period
LNPF lymph node permeability factor
LO linguo-occlusal; love object
LOA leave of absence; left anterior oblique view (of the heart); left occipitoanterior (position of fetus)
LOC liquid organic compound
lo cal low calorie (diet)
lo calc low calcium (diet)
loc cit *loco citato* (L) in the place quoted
loc dol *loco dolenti* (L) to the painful spot
log logarithm
log$_e$ logarithm to the base e

log₁₀ logarithm to the base 10

LOL left occipitolateral (position of fetus)

LOM limitation of movement or motion

LOMSA left otitis media suppurative acute

LOMSCh left otitis media suppurative chronic

long longitudinal; *longus* (L) long

LOP leave on pass; left occipitoposterior (position of fetus)

LOPS length of patient stay

lord lordosis(-otic)

LOS length of stay; Licentiate in Obstetrical Science

LOT left occipitotransverse (position of fetus)

lot *lotio* (L) lotion

LP laboratory procedure; laryngeal-pharyngeal; latent period; light perception; linguopulpal; lipoprotein; lower power (with reference to microscopy); low pressure; lumbar puncture

L/P lactate/pyruvate (ratio); lymphocyte/polymorph (ratio)

LPAM L-phenylalanine mustard (melphalan)

LPC lysophosphatidylcholine

LPF leucocytosis-promoting factor; low-power field

LPH left posterior hemiblock; lipotrophic pituitary hormone (lipotrophin)

LPL lamina propria lymphocytes; lipoprotein lipase

LPN Licensed Practical Nurse

LPO lobus parolfactorius

LpOH lysopine dehydrogenase

lps litres per second

lpw lumens per watt

LQ longevity quotient; lordosis quotient; lowest quadrant

LR laboratory report; latency relaxation; lateral rectus (muscle)

LRC lower rib cage

LRCP Licentiate of the Royal College of Physicians

LRCP&SI Licentiate of the Royal College of Physicians and Surgeons, Ireland

LRCS Licentiate of the Royal College of Surgeons

LRCSE Licenciate of the Royal College of Surgeons, Edinburgh

LRCSI Licentiate of the Royal College of Surgeons, Ireland

LRD living related donor

LRF latex and resorcinol formaldehyde; liver residue

factor; luteinizing hormone-releasing factor
LRH luteinizing hormone-releasing hormone
LRL Lunar Receiving Laboratory
LRR labyrinthine righting reflex
LRSF lactating rat serum factor
LRT lower respiratory tract
LRTI lower respiratory tract illness or infection
LS lateral suspensor; left sacrum; left side; leiomyosarcoma; Licentiate in Surgery; Life Science; liminal sensation; lumbosacral; lymphosarcoma
L/S lactase/sucrase ratio; lecithin/sphingomyelin ratio
LSA left sacroanterior (position of fetus); lichen sclerosis et atrophicus
LSB left sternal border
LSC left-side colon cancer; liquid scintillation counting
LScA left scapuloanterior (position of fetus)
LScP left scapuloposterior (position of fetus)
LSCS lower segment Caesarean section
LSD least significant difference; lysergic acid diethylamide (lysergide)
LSF lymphocyte-stimulating factor
LSH lymphocyte-stimulating hormone (factor)
LSHTM London School of Hygiene and Tropical Medicine
LSI large scale integrated (circuit)
LSK liver, spleen, kidneys
LSL left sacrolateral (position of fetus)
LSM lymphocyte separation medium; lysergic acid morpholide
LSO lateral superior olive (of the brain)
LSP left sacroposterior (position of fetus)
LSp life span
LSSA lipid-soluble secondary antioxidant
LST left sacrotransverse (position of fetus)
LSU lactose-saccharose-urea (agar)
LSWA large-amplitude, slow-wave activity
LT heat-labile enterotoxin; leukotriene; low temperature; lymphotoxin
lt left; low tension
LTA lipoate transacetylase; lipoteichoic acid
LTAS lead tetra-acetate Schiff
LTB laryngotracheal bronchitis
LTC leukotriene C; long-term care
LTD leukotriene D
ltd limited

LTE   leukotriene E

LTF   lipotropic factor; lymphocyte transforming factor

LTH   low-temperature holding (pasteurization); luteo-trophic hormone

LTP   long-term potentiation

LTPP   lipothiamide-pyrophosphate

LTR   large terminal repeats (genetics); long terminal repeats (virology)

LTT   lymphocyte transformation test

LTW   Leydig cell tumour of Wistar rats

LU   left upper

LUE   left upper extremity

Lues I   primary syphilis

Lues II   secondary syphilis

Lues III   tertiary syphilis

LUL   left upper eyelid; left upper lobe (of lung)

LUO   left ureteral orifice

LUOQ   left upper outer quadrant

LUQ   left upper quadrant (of abdomen)

lut   *luteum* (L) yellow

LV   *Lactobacillus viridescens;* left ventricle; live vaccine

Lv   leave

LVAD   left ventricular assist device

LVED   left ventricular end diastolic

LVEDD   left ventricle end-diastolic dimension

LVEDP   left ventricular end-diastolic pressure

LVEDV   left ventricular end-diastolic volume

LFEF   left ventricular ejection fraction

LVETI   left ventricular ejection time index

LVF   left ventricular failure

LVH   left ventricular hypertrophy

LVLG   left ventrolateral gluteal (site of injection)

LVN   Licensed Visiting Nurse; Licensed Vocational Nurse

LVS   left ventricular strain

LVSW   left ventricular stroke work

LVSWI   left ventricular stroke work index

LVT   lysine vasotonin

LVV   left ventricular volume

L&W   living and well

L-10-W   laevulose (10%) in water

LWCT   Lee-White clotting time

LXT   left exotopia

LY   lactoalbumin-yeastolate (media)

ly   langley (unit of sun's heat)

lym lymphocyte
lymph lymphocyte
lymphos lymphocytes
LYP lactose, yeast, peptone (agar)
Lys lysine
lytes electrolytes
LZM lysozyme

M

M *macerare* (L) macerate; male; malignant (with reference to tumours); married; masculine; mass; massage; maternally contributing (genetics); matrix; mature; maximal, maximum; mean (arithmetic); median; mediator (chemical, released in the tissues); medical; medicine; mega (prefix) (SI); memory (associative); *mentum* (L) chin; *meridies* (L) noon; mesial; metabolite; methotrexate; *Micrococcus; mille* (L) thousand; *misce* (L) mix; *mistura* (L) mixture; *mitte* (L) send; molar (solution); molar (tooth, permanent); molecular weight; Monday; monkey; morphine; *mortis* (L) death; mother; motile (with reference to bacteria); mucoid (with reference to bacterial colonies); murmur (heart); muscle; *mutitas* (L) dullness; myopia

m *manipulus* (L) handful; melts at (when followed by a figure denoting temperature); metre (SI); milli (prefix) (SI); minim; minute; molar (tooth, deciduous); murmur

μ micro (prefix) (SI); micrometre; mu

m- meta- (in chemical formulas); prefix denoting meso-position

M_1, M_2, M_3 Slight, marked, and absolute dullness (auscultation)

M_1 mitral (first) sound

M_2 dose per square metre of body surface

M/3 middle third (long bones)

MA Master of Arts; menstrual age; mental age; mentum anterior; meter angle; microagglutination; milliampere

MAA macroaggregated albumin; Medical Assistance to the Aged; monarticular arthritis

MAAGB Medical Artists Association of Great Britain

MABP mean arterial blood pressure

MAC MacConkey agar; malignancy associated changes; maximal allowable concentration; maximal allowable cost; Medical Alert Center; midarm circumference

mac *macerare* (L) macerate

m accur *misce accuratissime* (L) mix very intimately

macer *macera* (L) macerate

MAD methylandrostenediol (methandriol); mind-altering drug; myoadenylate deaminase

MAE Medical Air Evacuation

MAF macrophage activating factor; macrophage agglutinating factor; minimum audible field; movement after-effect

Mag magnesium

mag magnification; *magnus* (L) large

Magic microprobe analysis generalized intensity corrections

magn *magnus* (L) large

MAKA major karyotypic abnormality

MAL midaxillary line; malfunction

Mal malate

Mal-BSA maleated bovine serum albumin

MALIMET Master List of Medical Indexing Terms (EMBASE thesaurus)

M+Am compound myopic astigmatism

MAMA monoclonal anti-malignin antibody

ma-min milliampere-minute

MAN magnocellular nucleus (of anterior neostratum)

man *mane* (L) morning; *manipulus* (L) a handful

mand mandible

manifest manifestation

manip *manipulus* (L) a handful

man pr *mane primo* (L) early in the morning

manu manufacture

MAO Master of the Art of Obstetrics; monoamine oxidase

MAOI monoamine oxidase inhibitor

MAOT Member of the Association of Occupational Therapists

MAP mean arterial pressure; Medical Audit Program; mercapturic acid pathway; minimum audible pressure; muscle action potential

MAR margin; minimal angle resolution

MAS Medical Advisory Service; milliampere-second

mas masculine

MASA Medical Association of South Africa

masc masculine
MASER microwave amplification by stimulated emission of radiation
MASH Mobile Army Surgical Hospital
MASP microaerophilous stationary phase
mas pil *massa pilularum* (L) a pill mass
mass massage
MAST medical antishock trousers
mast mastoid
MASU Mobile Army Surgical Unit
MAT manual arts therapist; mature, maturity
math mathematics(-ical)
MATRIS Medical Manpower and Training Information Service (Brit)
matut *matutinus* (L) in the morning
max maxilla; maximum
MB buccal margin; Marsh-Bender factor (an ATP inhibitor in muscle tissue); *Medicinae Baccalaureus* (L) Bachelor of Medicine; mesiobuccal; methyl bromide; methylene blue
mb *misce bene* (L) mix well
MBAC Member of the British Association of Chemists
MBC maximum breathing capacity; methylthymol blue complex
MBD minimal brain dysfunction
MB factor Marsh-Bender factor
MBH medial basal hypothalamus
MBH$_2$ methylene blue reduced
MBL Marine Biological Laboratory (Woods Hole, Mass); menstrual blood loss
MBLA methylbenzyl linoleic acid
MBM mineral basal medium
MBNOA Member British Naturopathic and Osteopathic Association
MBO mesiobucco-occlusal
MBP mean blood pressure; melitensis, bovine, porcine; mesiobuccopulpal; myelin basic protein
MBR methylene blue reduced
MBRT methylene blue reduction time
MC *Magister Chirurgiae* (L) Master of Surgery; mast cell; Medical Corps; Merkel cell; mesiocervical; metacarpal; mitomycin; mitochondrial complementation; mixed cryoglobulinaemia; monkey cells; myocarditis
M-C Medico-Chirurgical; mineralocorticoid (with reference to adrenal cortical hormones)

M&C morphine and cocaine
Mc megacycle
mC millicoulomb (SI)
MCA major coronary arteries; Manufacturing Chemists Association; Maternity Center Association
MCAT Medical College Admission Test
m caute *misce caute* (L) mix cautiously
MCB membranous cytoplasmic bodies
McB McBurney's point
MCBM muscle capillary basement membrane
MCC marked cocontraction
McC McCarthy (panendoscope); McCoy antibodies
MCCNU methyl-CCNU (semustine)
MCCU Mobile Coronary Care Unit
MCD mean corpuscular diameter; metacarpal cortical density; minimal changes disease; multiple carboxylase deficiency
mcd millicuries destroyed
MCF medium corpuscular fragility
mcg microgram
MCGN mixed cryoglobulinaemia associated with glomerulonephritis
MCH Maternal and Child Health; mean corpuscular haemoglobin
MCh *Magister Chirurgiae* (L) Master of Surgery
mc h millicurie hour
MCHC mean corpuscular haemoglobin concentration
MChD Master of Dental Surgery
MChir Master in Surgery
MChOrth Master of Orthopaedic Surgery
MChOtol Master of Oto-Rhino-Laryngological Surgery
MCHR Medical Committee for Human Rights
MCHS Maternal and Child Health Service
MChS Member of the Society of Chiropodists
MCi megacurie (SI)
mCi millicurie (SI)
MCKD multicystic kidney disease
MCL midclavicular line; modified chest lead; most comfortable loudness (audiometry)
MClSci Master of Clinical Science
MCommH Master of Community Health
mcoul millicoulomb
μcoul microcoulomb
MCP Medical College of Pennsylvania; Medical Continuation Pay (Military); metacarpophalangeal

MCPA Member of the College of Pathologists, Australasia

MCPH metacarpophalangeal

MCPS Member of the College of Physicians & Surgeons

Mcps megacycles per second

MCR Medical Corps Reserve; metabolic clearance rate

MCRA Member of the College of Radiologists, Australasia

MCSP Member of the Chartered Society of Physiotherapy

MCT mean cell thickness; mean circulation time; medium chain triglyceride; medullary cancer of the thyroid; multiple compressed tablet

MCTD mixed connective tissue disease

MCU Malaria Control Unit (Army)

MCV mean corpuscular volume

MCZ Museum of Comparative Zoology (Harvard Univ)

MD main duct; malic dehydrogenase; manic-depressive; mean deviation; Medical Department; *Medicinae Doctor* (L) Doctor of Medicine; mentally deficient; mesiodistal; mitral disease; monocular deprivation; muscular dystrophy; myocardial disease

md median

MDA *mento-dextra anterior* (L) right mentoanterior (position of fetus); monohydroascorbate; motor discriminative acuity; Muscular Dystrophy Association

MDBDF March of Dimes Birth Defect Foundation

MDBK Madin-Darby bovine kidney (cells)

MDCK Madin-Darby-canine kidney (cell line)

MDD Doctor of Dental Medicine

MDentSc Master of Dental Science

MDF myocardial depressant factor

MDH malic dehydrogenase; medullary dorsal horn

m dict *more dictu* (L) in the manner directed

mdn median

MDNB metadinitrobenzene

MDOPA alpha-methyl-dopa

MDP *mento-dextra posterior* (L) right mentoposterior (position of fetus)

MDQ minimum detectable quantity

MDR minimum daily requirement

MDS Master of Dental Surgery

MDT *mento-dextra transversa* (L) right mentotransverse (position of fetus)

MDU Medical Defence Union (Brit)

MDV Marek's disease virus
ME maximum effort; median eminence (of hypothalamus); Medical Examiner; mercaptoethanol; metabolizable energy; middle ear; mouse epithelial (cells)
M/E myeloid/erythrocyte (ratio)
Me methyl (CH_3)
MEA Medical Exhibition Association; mercaptoethyl amine; multiple endocrine adenomas
meas measure(ment)
MeB Medical Board; methylene blue
MEC middle ear cells; minimum effective concentration
mec meconium
Mecano mechanotherapy
Me-CCNU methyl-CCNU (semustine)
mech mechanical
MED median erythrocyte diameter; medical; medicine; minimal effective dose; minimal erythema dose
med medial, median; medical; medication; medicine, medical; medium (bacteriology)
MEDEX *médecin extension* (F) extension of the physician (with reference to recruitment program)
MEDICO Medical International Cooperation
MEDICS Medical Information and Career Service (Brit)
MEDLARS Medical Literature Analysis and Retrieval System (database)
MEDLINE An on-line segment of MEDLARS
MEDScD Doctor of Medical Science
MedSurg medicine and surgery
Med Tech Medical Technician; Medical Technology (-ologist)
MEE methylethyl ether; middle ear effusion
MEF maximal expiratory flow; middle ear fluid; mid-expiratory flow; mouse embryo fibroblasts
MEG magnetoencephalogram
mEGB mouse epidermal growth factor
MEL metabolic equivalent level
MEM minimum essential medium
mem member
memb membrane
MEND Medical Education for National Defense
Menn Menninger
ment mental
MeOH methyl alcohol
MEP mean effective pressure; motor end-plate
MEPP miniature end-plate potential

mEq milliequivalent
MER ethamoxytriphetol (an anti-oestrogen); methanol-extracted residue
MERB Medical Examination and Review Board (DOD)
MES maintenance electrolyte solution; maximum electroshock seizure; morpholino-ethanesulphonic acid
Mesc mescaline
MeSH Medical Subject Headings (MEDLARS)
MET metabolic equivalent of the task; metastasis; mid-expiratory time
Met methionine
met metallic (with reference to chest sounds)
metab metabolism, metabolic
metaph metaphysics
metas metastasis(-stasize)
METH methicillin
Meth methedrine (methylamphetamine hydrochloride)
meth methyl
MeTHF methyltetrahydrofolic acid
M et n *mane et nocte* (L) morning and night
METS metabolic equivalents
m et sig *misce et signa* (L) mix and write a label
mev million electron volts
MF microscopic factor; mitogenic factor; mitotic figure; multiplying factor; mycosis fungoides; myelin figure; myofibrillar
M/F male to female (ratio)
Mf *Microfilaria*
mF millifarad (SI)
μF microfarad (SI)
MFA monofluoroacetate
MFCM Master, Faculty of Community Medicine
m-FC membrane faecal coli (broth)
MFD minimum fatal dose
mfd microfarad
MFG modified heat degraded gelatin
mfg manufacturing(-ed)
MFH malignant fibrous histiocytoma
MFHom Member of the Faculty of Homeopathy
MFID multielectrode flame ionization detector
M flac *membrana flaccida* (L) Shrapnell's membrane
MFOM Master, Faculty of Occupational Medicine
MFP myofascial pain
mfr manufacturer
MF sol merthiolate-formaldehyde (stock) solution

MFSS Medical Field Service School (Army)
MFST Medical Field Service Technician
MFT muscle function test
m ft *mistura fiat* (L) let a mixture be made
MG margin; menopausal gonadotrophin; mesiogingival; methylglucoside; myasthenia gravis
Mg magnesium
mg milligram (SI)
mg% milligrams per 100 ml
μg microgram (SI)
MGA melengestrol acetate
MGC minimal glomerular change nephrology
MGD mixed gonadal dysgenesis
mgd million gallons per day
MGDS Member in General Dental Surgery
mg-el milligram element
MGH Massachusetts General Hospital
mgh milligram-hour
mgm milligram
MGP marginal granulocyte pool
MGW magnesium sulphate, glycerine, water (enema)
MH malignant histiocytosis; malignant hyperpyrexia or hyperthermia; mammotrophic hormone (prolactin); marital history; Master Herbalist; medical history; melanophore hormone; menstrual history; mental health; murine hepatitis
M-H Mueller-Hinton (agar)
mH millihenry
MHA Mental Health Administration
MHb myohaemoglobin
MHBSS modified Hank's balanced salt solution
MHC major histocompatibility complex; Mental Health Care (Brit)
mhcb mean horizontal candle power
MHCS Mental Hygiene Consultation Service
MHCU Mental Health Care Unit
MHD magnetohydrodynamics; maintenance haemodialysis; Medical Holding Detachment; Mental Health Department; Mental Health Digest; minimum haemolytic dose
MHLC Multidimensional Health Locus of Control (diagnostic scale)
MHLS metabolic heat load simulator
MHP Mental Health Project
MHR major histocompatibility region; maximum heart

rate; methaemoglobin reductase

MHRI Mental Health Research Institute (Univ of Michigan)

MHS major histocompatibility system; malignant hypothermia susceptible (patients)

MHyg Master of Hygiene

MHz megahertz (SI)

MI medical inspection; melanophore index; menstrual induction; mesioincisal; metabolic index; migration inhibition; mitotic index; mitral incompetence; mitral insufficiency; myocardial infarction; myo-inositol

MIBiol Member of the Institute of Biology

MIBT methyl isatin-beta-thiosemicarbasone

MIC Medical Interfraternity Conference; microscopic findings in centrifugal urinary sediment; microscopy (-scopic); minimal inhibitory concentration; minimal isorrhoeic concentration

Microbiol microbiology

MICU Mobile Intensive Care Unit

MID mesioincisodistal; minimal inhibiting dose; minimum infective dose

mid middle

mid sag midsagittal

MIF melanocyte-stimulating hormone release-inhibiting factor; merthiolate-iodine-formaldehyde; mid-inspiratory flow; migration-inhibitory factor (for macrophages)

MIFR maximal inspiratory flow rate

MIg membrane immunoglobulin; malaria immunoglobulin; measles immunoglobulin

MIH Master of Industrial Health

MIKA minor karyotypic abnormalities

mil military

MIMS Medical Inventory Management System; Medical Information Management System; Monthly Index of Medical Specialities

MIN medial interlaminar nucleus

min mineral; *minimum* (L) a minim; minimum, minimal; minor; minute

MINA monoisonitrosoacetone

MINIA monkey intranuclear inclusion agent

MInstSP Member Institution of Sewage Purification

MIO minimal identifiable odour; motility indol ornithine (medium)

misc miscarriage; miscellaneous

MIST   Medical Information Service by Telephone

mist *mistura* (L) a mixture

MIT   Massachusetts Institute of Technology; miracidial immobilization test; mono-iodotyrosine

mit *mitte* (L) send

mit insuf mitral insufficiency

mitt *mitte* (L) send

mitte sang *mitte sanguinem* (L) bleed

mitt tal *mitte tales* (L) send such

mixt *mixture* (L) mixture

MJ   marijuana

MJI   Masters and Johnson Institute

MK   monkey kidney

MKB   megakaryoblast

mkg   metre kilogram

mks   metre-kilogram-second

ML   Licentiate in Medicine; Licentiate in Midwifery; lingual margin; mesiolingual; midline

M-L   Martin-Lewis (medium)

mL   millilambert

ml   millilitre (SI)

MLA   Medical Library Association; *mento-laeva anterior* (L) left mentoanterior (position of fetus)

MLa   mesiolabial

MLal   mesiolabioincisal

MLaP   mesiolabiopulpal

MLC   mixed leucocyte culture

MLCO   Member of the London College of Osteopathy

MLD   metachromatic leucodystrophy; minimal lethal dose

MLD 50   median lethal dose (radiation)

MLI   mesiolinguoincisal

MLO   mesiolinguo-occlusal

MLP   *mento-laeva posterior* (L) left mentoposterior (position of fetus); mesiolinguopulpal

MLS   median life span; median longitudinal section

MLT   median lethal time (radiation); Medical Laboratory Technician; *mento-laeva transversa* (L) left mento-transverse (position of fetus)

MLV   multilaminar vesicles; murine leukaemia virus

MLVSS   mixed liquor volatile suspended solids

MM   Major Medical (insurance); malignant melanoma; mucous membrane; myeloid metaplasia

mM   millimolar

mm   methylmalonyl (CoA mutase); millimetre; muscles

μm micrometre (micron) (SI)

MMA medical materials account (military); methylmalonic acid

MMATP methadone maintenance and aftercare treatment program

MMC migrating myoelectric complexes

MMD mass median diameter (of particles)

MMED Master of Medicine

MMEFR maximum mid-expiratory flow rate

MMF maximum mid-expiratory flow (rate); Member of the Medical Faculty

MMFR maximum mid-expiratory flow rate

MMG mean maternal glucose

mmHg millimetres of mercury

MMIS Medicade Management and Information System

MMLV Moloney murine leukaemia virus

mmm millimicron (nanometer)

MMPI Minnesota Multiphasic Personality Inventory

MMPNC Medical Maternal Program for Nuclear Casualties

mmpp millimetres partial pressure

MMR Mass Miniature Radiography; maternal mortality rate; measles, mumps, rubella; monomethylolrutin

MMS Master of Medical Science

MMSA Master of Midwifery, Society of Apothecaries

MMSc Master of Medical Science

mm st muscle strength

MMT manual muscle test

MMTV mouse mammary tumour virus

MMU Medical Maintenance Unit (Army); mercaptomethyl uracil

mmu millimass units

mμ millimicron (nanometre)

mμc millimicrocurie (nanocurie)

mμg millimicrogram (nanogram)

μl microlitre (SI)

μmg micromilligram

μmm micromillimetre

μμ micromicron (picometre)

μμc micromicrocurie (picocurie)

μμg micromicrogram (picogram)

MMWR Morbidity and Mortality Weekly Report (CDC)

MN Master of Nursing; mononuclear (leucocyte); motor neuron; multinodular; myoneural

M-N motility nitrate (medium)

Mn manganese
mN millinormal
MND minimum necrosing dose; motor neuron disease
mng morning
MNJ myoneural junction
MNL mononuclear leukocytes
MO manually operated; Master of Obstetrics; Master of Osteopathy; Medical Officer; mesio-occlusal; mineral oil; minute output (of heart); mono-oxygenase
Mo mode; molybdenum
mo month
mob mobilization
mobil mobility
MOC maximum oxygen consumption
MOD maturity onset diabetes; Medical Officer of the Day; Medicine, Osteopathy, and Dentistry; mesio-occlusodistal
mod moderate
mod praesc *modo praescripto* (L) in the manner prescribed or as directed
MOF marine oxidation/fermentation (medium); multiple organ failure
MO&G Master of Obstetrics and Gynaecology
MOH Medical Officer of Health
MΩ megohm (SI)
$\mu\Omega$ microhm (SI)
mol molecule(-ular)
mol/l molecules per litre
moll *mollis* (L) soft
mol wt molecular weight
MOM milk of magnesia
mon monocyte
Mono mononucleosis
mono monocyte
MOOW Medical Officer of the Watch
MOP medical out-patient
MOPP mustine, oncovin (vincristine), procarbazine, and prednisone
MOPV monovalent oral poliovirus vaccine
MOR Medical Officer Report (Navy); morphine
MORC Medical Officers Reserve Corps
mor dict *more dicto* (L) in the manner directed
morph morphology(-ological)
mor sol *more solito* (L) in the usual manner
mortal mortality

mos months

mOsm milliosmole

MOTT mycobateria other than tubercle (bacilli)

MOUS multiple occurrences of unexplained symptoms

MOX moxalactam (latamoxef sodium)

MP medial payment; melphalan and prednisone; menstrual period; mentum posterior; mercaptopurine; mesiopulpal; metacarpophalangeal; metatatarsophalangeal; methylprednisolone sodium succinate; mucopolysaccharide; mycoplasmal pneumonia

mp melting point

MPA Medical Procurement Agency; medroxyprogesterone acetate (Depo-Provera)

MPB male pattern baldness

MPC maximum permissible concentration; minimum protozoacidal contamination

MPCU maximum permissible concentration of unidentified radionucleotides

MPD maximum permissible dose; myofacial pain dysfunction

MPE maximum possible error

MPGM monophosphoglycerate mutase

MPGN membranous proliferative glomerulonephritis

MPH Master of Public Health; milk protein hydrolysate

mph miles per hour

MPharm Master in Pharmacy

MPI maximal permitted intake; maximum point of impulse; multiphasic personality inventory; myocardial perfusion imaging

MPL maximum permissible level; melphalan

MPM malignant papillary mesothelioma; multipurpose meal

MPN most probable number

MPO myeloperoxidase

MPP Medical Personnel Pool

MPPT methylprednisolone pulse therapy

MPR marrow production rate

MPS Member of the Pharmaceutical Society; Microbial Profile System; mononuclear phagocyte system; movement produced stimuli; mucopolysaccharide; multiphasic screening

MPsyMed Master of Psychological Medicine

MPU Medical Practitioners Union

MPV mean platelet volume

MR may repeat; measles-rubella; medial rectus (muscle);

Medical Record; mentally retarded; metabolic rate; methyl red; mitral regurgitation

mR milliroentgen

μR microroentgen

MRA Medical Record Administrator

MRAA Mental Retardation Association of America

MRACGP Member of the Royal Australasian College of General Practice

MRACO Member of the Royal Australasian College of Ophthalmologists

MRACP Member of Royal Australasian College of Physicians

MRACR Member of the Royal Australasian College of Radiologists

MRad Master of Radiology

mrad millirad

MRANZCP Member of the Royal Australian and New Zealand College of Psychiatrists

MRBC monkey red blood cells

MRBF mean renal blood flow

MRC Medical Registration Council; Medical Research Council; Medical Reserve Corps; methylrosaniline chloride (crystal violet)

MRCGP Member of the Royal College of General Practitioners

MRCI Medical Registration Council of Ireland; Medical Research Council of Ireland

MRCOG Member of the Royal College of Obstetricians and Gynaecologists

MRCP Member of the Royal College of Physicians

MCRPA Member of the Royal College of Pathologists of Australia

MRCPath Member of the Royal College of Pathologists

MRCPE Member of the Royal College of Physicians of Edinburgh

MRCP(Glasg) Member of the Royal College of Physicians and Surgeons of Glasgow *qua* Physician

MRCPI Member of the Royal College of Physicians of Ireland

MRCPsych Member of the Royal College of Psychiatrists

MRCS Member of the Royal College of Surgeons

MRCSE Member of the Royal College of Surgeons of Edinburgh

MRCSI Member of the Royal College of Surgeons in Ireland

MRCVS Member of the Royal College of Veterinary Surgeons

MRD minimal residual disease; minimum reaction dose

mrd millirutherford

mrem milliroentgen equivalent man

mrep milliroentgen equivalent physical

MRF midbrain reticular formation; MSH releasing factor; Müllerian regression factor

MRFT modified rapid fermentation test

MRH MSH-releasing hormone

MRHA mannose-resistant haemagglutination

mrhm milliroentgen per hour at one metre

MRI Medical Research Institute; Member of the Royal Institution; Mental Research Institute; moderate renal insufficiency

MRIF MSH release inhibiting factor

MRIPHH Member of the Royal Institute of Public Health and Hygiene

MRL Medical Record Librarian; Medical Research Laboratory (Navy and Air Force)

mRNA messenger ribonucleic acid

MRO muscle receptor organ

MROD Medical Research and Operations Directorate (NASA)

MRP Medical Reimbursement Plan; Members Retirement Plan (of AMA)

MRR marrow release rate

MRS Medical Receiving Station

MRSH Member of the Royal Society of Health

MRT muscle response test

MRU Mass Radiography Unit; minimal reproductive units (bacteriology)

MRV minute respiratory volume; mixed respiratory vaccine

MRVP methyl red, Voges-Proskauer (medium)

MS complex of substrate and activating metal ion; maladjustment score; mass spectrometry; Master of Science; Master of Surgery; Medical Services (Navy); medical supplies; Medical Survey; mentally retarded; mitral stenosis; Mobile Surgery (Brit); modal sensitivity; molar solution; Mongolian spot; morphine sulphate; motile sperm; multiple sclerosis; muscle shortening; muscle strength; musculoskeletal

Ms manuscript

ms millisecond (SI)

μs   microsecond (SI)
MS-222   tricaine methane sulphonate
MSA   manitol salt agar (plate); Medical Services Administration; mine safety appliance
MSAA   multiple sclerosis-associated agent
MSB   Martius Scarlet Blue
MsB   Master of Science in Bacteriology
MSBLA   mouse-specific B lymphocyte antigen
MSC   Medical Service Corps; Medical Specialist Corps; Medical Staff Corps (Brit)
MSc   Master of Science
MScD   Doctor of Medical Science; Doctor of Science in Medicine; Master of Dental Science
MScMed   Master of Medical Science
MScN   Master of Science in Nursing
mscp   mean spherical candle power
MSDC   Mass Spectrometry Data Centre (UK)
MSE   medical support equipment
mse   mean square error
MSEA   Medical Society Executives Association
msec   millisecond
μ**sec**   microsecond
MSES   medical school environmental stress
MSF   macrophage spreading factor
MSG   monosodium glutamate
MSH   melanocyte-stimulating hormone; melanophore-stimulating hormone (intermedin)
MSH-IF   MSH-inhibiting factor
MSHyg   Master of Science in Hygiene
MSKCC   Memorial Sloan-Kettering Cancer Centre
MSKP   Medical Sciences Knowledge Profile
MSL   midsternal line
MSM   Master of Medical Science; mineral salts medium; medial superior olive (of the brain)
MSN   Master of Science in Nursing
MSPGN   mesangial proliferative glomerulonephritis
MSPH   Master of Science in Public Health
MSPhar   Master of Science in Pharmacy
MSPS   myocardial stress perfusion scintigraphy
MS in Rad   Master of Science in Radiology
MSR   Member of the Society of Radiographers
MSRG   Member of the Society for Remedial Gymnasts
MSRPP   multidimensional scale for rating psychiatric patients
MSS   massage; Medical Service School (Air Force);

Medical Superintendents' Society; mental status schedule; motion sickness susceptibility; mucus-stimulating substance

Mss manuscripts

MSSc Master of Sanitary Science

MSSE Master of Science in Sanitary Engineering

MSSR Medical Society for the Study of Radiesthesia

MSSVD Medical Society for the Study of Venereal Diseases

MST mean survival time; mean swell time (botulism test)

MSTh mesothorium

MSU medical studies unit; mid-stream urine specimen

MSUD maple syrup urine disease

MSurg Master of Surgery

MSV maximal sustained level of ventilation; murine sarcoma virus

MSW Master of Social Welfare; Master of Social Work; Medical Social Worker

MSWYE modified sea water yeast extract (agar)

MT empty; malaria therapy; mammary tumour; Medical Technologist; membrana tympani; metatarsal; microtome; microtubule; music therapy

M-T macroglobulin-trypsin complex

MT6 mercaptomerin

MTA Medical Technical Assistant

MT(ASCP) Registered Medical Technologist (American Society of Clinical Pathologists)

MTC medical test cabinet; Medical Training Center; medullary thyroid carcinoma; mitomycin C

MTD maximally tolerated dose; Midwife Teacher's Diploma

mtd *mitte tales doses* (L) send such doses

MTF Medical Treatment Faculty

MTH mithramycin

MTLP metabolic toxaemia of late pregnancy

MTM modified Thayer-Martin medium

MTO Medical Transport Officer

MTOC microtubule organizing centre; mitotic organizing centre

MTP metatarsophalangeal; microtubule protein

MTR Meinicke turbidity reaction; Mental Treatment Rules

MTT mean transit time (*see* TT)

MTU methylthiouracil

M tuberc *Mycobacterium tuberculosis*

MTV   mammary tumour virus
MTX   methotrexate
MU   mouse unit (with reference to gonadotrophins)
Mu   Mache unit (with reference to radium emanations)
mu   micron (μm)
MUC   maximum urinary concentration
muc   *mucilago* (L) mucilage
mult   multiple
MuLV   murine leukaemia virus
MUO   myocardiopathy of unknown origin
MurNAc   N-acetylmuramate
MURC   measurable undesirable respiratory contaminants
musc   muscle, muscular
MUWU   mouse uterine weight unit
MV   *Medicus Veterinarius* (L) veterinary physician; microvilli; microwave; minute volume; mitral value
mV   millivolt (SI)
μV   microvolt (SI)
MVA   mitral valve area
MVB   multivesicular body
MVD   Doctor of Veterinary Medicine
MVE   Murray Valley encephalitis
MVLS   mandibular vestibulolingual sulcoplasty
MVMT   movement
MVP   mitral valve prolapse
MVPP   mustine, vinblastine, procarbazine, prednisone
MVPS   mitral valve prolapse syndrome
MVR   mitral valve replacement
MVRI   mixed vaccine, respiratory infections
MVV   maximum voluntary ventilation
MW   molecular weight
μW   microwatt (SI)
MX   matrix
My   myopia
my   mayer (unit of heat capacity)
Myco   *Mycobacterium*
Mycol   mycology
Myel   myelocyte
myel   myelin(ated)
MyG   myasthenia gravis
MYS   myasthenic syndrome
MZ   mantle zone; monozygotic
MZA   monozygotic twins raised apart
MZT   monozygotic twins raised together

N

N nasal; negative; negro; nerve; neurology(-ologist); neuropathy; newton (SI); nicotinamide; nitrogen; nodules; non-malignant (with reference to tumours); Nonne (globulin test); normal (with reference to solutions); normal (with reference to structure and functioning of organs); number

n born; symbol for index of refraction; haploid chromosome number (2n equals diploid number); nano (prefix) (SI); *naris* (L) nostril; nasal; *natus* (L) born; neuter; neutron; neutron dosage (unit of); number; symbol (chemical) for normal (i.e. containing an unbranched chain of carbon atoms)

^{15}N radioactive nitrogen

NI, NII, etc cranial nerves No 1, No 2, etc

NA Narcotics Anonymous; neuraminidase; neutrophil antibody; nicotinic acid; Nomina Anatomica; noradrenaline; nucleic acid; nucleus ambiguus; numerical aperture; nurse's aide; Nursing Assistant; Nursing Auxiliary (Brit)

Na Avogadro's number; *natrium* (L) sodium

^{24}Na radioactive sodium

NAA naphthaleneacetic acid; nicotinic acid amide; no apparent abnormalities

NAACLS National Accrediting Agency for Clinical Laboratory Sciences

NAACOG Nurses Association of the American College of Obstetricians and Gynecologists

NAACP neoplasia, allergy, Addison's disease, collagen vascular disease, and parasites

NAAFA National Association to Aid Fat Americans

NAAP N-acetyl-4-amino-phenazone

NAB novarsenobenzene (neoarsphenamine)

NABP National Association of Boards of Pharmacy

NAC N-acetyl-L-cysteine; National Asthma Center; Noise Advisory Council

NACDS North American Clinical Dermatologic Society

NACED National Advisory Council on the Employment of the Disabled

NACOR National Advisory Committee on Radiation

NAD nicotinamide-adenine dinucleotide; no acute distress; no appreciable disease; nothing abnormal detected

NADA New Animal Drug Applications

NADP nicotinamide-adenine-dinucleotide phosphate
NADPH NADP (reduced form)
Na$_e$ exchangeable body sodium
NAF National Amputation Foundation; National Ataxia Foundation
NAG non-agglutinating
NAHCS National Association of Health Career Schools
NAHG National Association of Humanistic Gerontology
NAHI National Athletic Health Institute
NAHPA National Association of Hospital Purchasing Agents
NAHSA National Association for Hearing and Speech Action
NAHSE National Association of Health Services Executives
NAHU National Association of Health Underwriters
NAI non-accidental injury
NAM natural actomyosins
NAMCS National Ambulatory Medical Care Survey
NAMH National Association for Mental Health
NAMRU Navy Medical Reserve Unit
NAMS National Ambient Air Monitoring Stations; Nurses and Army Medical Specialists
NANA N-acetyl neuraminic acid
NANBH non-A, non-B hepatitis
NAOO National Association of Optometrists and Opticians
NAOP National Alliance for Optional Parenthood
NAP nasion pogonion (angle of convexity); neutrophil alkaline phosphatase; nucleic acid phosphorus
NAPA N-acetyl-*p*-aminophenol (paracetamol)
NAPCA National Air Pollution Control Administration
NaPG sodium pregnanediol glucuronide
NAPH naphthyl
NAPN National Association of Physicians' Nurses
NAPNAP National Association of Pediatric Nurses Associates and Practitioners
NAPNES National Association for Practical Nurse Education and Service
NAPPH National Association of Private Psychiatric Hospitals
NAPT National Association for the Prevention of Tuberculosis
NAR nasal airway resistance
NARA Narcotics Addict Rehabilitation Act; National

Association of Recovered Alcoholics
NARAL National Abortion Rights Action League
NARC narcotic; narcotics officer; National Association for Retarded Children
narco narcotics hospital; narcotics officer; narcotics treatment center
NARD National Association of Retail Druggists
NARMC Naval Aerospace and Regional Medical Center
NARMH National Association for Rural Mental Health
NARS National Acupuncture Research Society
NAS nasal; National Academy of Sciences; National Association of Sanitarians; no added salt
NASA National Aeronautics and Space Administration
NASE National Association for the Study of Epilepsy
NASEAN National Association for State Enrolled Assistant Nurses
NASM Naval Aviation School of Medicine
NASMV National Association on Standard Medical Vocabulary
NAT N-acetyltransferase; natal
Nat national; native; natural
Natr *natrium* (L) sodium
NB newborn; *nota bene* (L) note well, take notice
NBC non-battle casualty
NBI no bone injury; non-battle injuries
NBM nothing by mouth
NBME National Board of Medical Examiners
NBRT National Board for Respiratory Therapy
NBS National Bureau of Standards
NBT nitro blue tetrazolium
NBTNF newborn, term, normal, female
NBTNM newborn, term, normal, male
NBTS National Blood Transfusion Service
NC neural crest; nitrocellulose; no change; nose cone; Nurse Corps
nc nanocurie
NCA National Certification Agency for Medical Lab Personnel; National Council on Aging; National Council on Alcoholism; neurocirculatory asthenia; nonspecific cross-reacting antigen
NCAE National Center for Alcohol Education
NCAMI National Committee Against Mental Illness
N-CAP Nurses Coalition for Action in Politics
NCCDC National Center for Chronic Disease Control
NCCDS National Cooperative Crohn's Disease Study

NCCIP National Center for Clinical Infant Programs

NCCLVP National Coordinating Committee on Large Volume Parenterals

NCCPA National Commission on Certification of Physician's Assistants

NCCU Newborn Convalescent Care Unit

NCD National Commission on Diabetes; National Council on Drugs; normal childhood disorders

NCDA National Council on Drug Abuse

NCE new chemical entities; nonconvulsive epilepsy

NCF neutrophil chemotactic factor

NCFA Narcolepsy and Catalepsy Foundation of America

NCGS National Cooperative Gallstone Study

NCHC National Council of Health Centers

NCHCT National Center for Health Care Technology

NCHMHHSO National Coalition of Hispanic Mental Health and Human Services Organizations

NCHS National Center for Health Statistics

NCHSR National Center for Health Services Research

NCI National Cancer Institute

nCi nanocurie (SI)

NCIB National Collection of Industrial Bacteria

NCL National Chemical Laboratory; neuronal ceroid lipofuscinosis

NCMH National Committee for Mental Health

NCMHI National Clearinghouse for Mental Health Information (HHS)

NCMI National Committee against Mental Illness

NCN National Council of Nurses

NCP noncollagen protein

NCPE noncardiac pulmonary edema

NCR nuclear-cytoplasmic ratio

NCRND National Committee for Research in Neurological Diseases

NCRPM National Committee on Radiation Protection and Measurements

NCRV National Committee for Radiation Victims

NCSC National Council of Senior Citizens

NCSN National Council for School Nurses

NCT neural crest tumour

NCTC National Collection of Type Cultures

ND natural death; Naval Dispensary; neoplastic disease; nervous debility; neutral density; Newcastle disease; New Drug; normal delivery; not detected; not determined; not diagnosed; Nursing Doctorate

N&D nodular and diffuse (lymphoma)
N$_d$ refractive index (symbol for)
Nd neodymium; number of dissimilar (matches)
NDA National Dental Association; new drug application; no detectable activity
NDC Naval Dental Clinic; National Drug Code
NDCR National Drug Code Directory
NDDG National Diabetes Data Group
NDE near death experience
NDGA nordihydro-guaiaretic acid
NDI nephrogenic diabetes insipidus
NDIR nondispersive infrared analyser
NDM New Dimensions in Medicine
NDS Naval Dental School
NDSB Narcotic Drugs Supervisory Board
NDT non-destructive testing
NDTA National Dental Technicians Association
NDTI National Disease and Therapeutic Index
NDV Newcastle disease virus
NE National Emergency; nerve excitability (test); neural excitation; neurological examination; no effect; norepinephrine; not enlarged; not examined
Ne neon
nebul *nebula* (L) a spray
NEC necrotizing enterocolitis; not elsewhere classified
NECHI Northeastern Consortium for Health Information
NECP New England College of Pharmacy
NED no evidence of disease; no expiration date; normal equivalent deviation
NEEP negative and expiratory pressure
NEFA non-esterified fatty acid
neg negative (symbol: −); negro
NEHE Nurses for Environmental Health Education
nem *Nährungsteinheit Milch* (Ger) nutritional unit milk
nema nematode (threadworm)
NEMCH New England Medical Center Hospitals
NEMD nonspecific esophageal motor dysfunction
neo negative expiratory pressure; neoarsphenamine
NEP negative expiratory pressure; nephrology
NERHL Northeastern Radiological Health Laboratory
nerv nervous
NES not elsewhere specified
NESP Nurse Education Support Program
NET nasoendotracheal tube; norethisterone

n et m *nocte et mane* (L) night and morning
ne tr s num *ne tradas sine nummo* (L) do not deliver unless paid
Neurol neurology
Neuropath neuropathology(-ologist)
Neuro-Surg neurosurgeon(-surgery)
neut neuter; neutral
NEX nose to ear to xiphoid
NEY neomycin egg yolk agar
NF National Formulary; nephritic factor; neurofibromatosis; neutral fraction; noise factor; none found; nonfiltered; nonwhite female; normal flow
NFB National Foundation for the Blind; nonfermenting bacteria
NFC National Fertility Center; not favourably considered
NFD neurofibrillary degeneration
NFIC National Foundation for Ileitis and Colitis
NFID National Foundation for Infectious Diseases
NFIP National Foundation for Infantile Paralysis
NFLPN National Federation of Licensed Practical Nurses
NFMD National Foundation for Muscular Dystrophy
NFME National Fund for Medical Education
NFND National Foundation for Neuromuscular Diseases
NFNID National Foundation for Non-Invasive Diagnostics
NFS National Fertility Study
NFT neurofibrillary tangle
NFTD normal full term delivery
NG nasogastric; new growth; no good
ng nanogram (SI)
NGC nucleus reticularis gigantocellularis
NGF nerve growth factor
NGR narrow gauze roll
NGSA nerve growth stimulating activity
NGU non-gonococcal urethritis
NH Naval Hospital; nursing home
NH₃ ammonia
NHA National Health Association; National Hearing Association; National Hemophilia Association
NHANES National Health and Nutritional Examination Survey
NHAS National Hearing Aid Association
NHBPCC National High Blood Pressure Coordinating

Committee
NHDS National Hospital Discharge Survey
NHF National Health Federation
NHG normal human globulin
NHI National Health Insurance; National Heart Institute
NHLBI National Heart, Lung and Blood Institute
NHLI National Heart and Lung Institute
NHMRC National Health and Medical Research Council
NHP New Health Practitioners (Nurse Practitioners and Physician's Assistants); normal human pooled plasma
NHPF National Health Policy Forum
NHRC National Health Research Center
NHS National Health Service; normal human serum
NHSAS National Health Service Audit Staff (Brit)
NHSR National Hospital Service Reserve
NI neurological improvement; no information; Noise Index
Ni nickel
NIA National Institute of Aging; no information available; Nutrition Institute of America
NIAAA National Institute on Alcohol Abuse and Alcoholism
NIADDK National Institute of Arthritis, Diabetes, and Digestive and Kidney Diseases
NIAID National Institute of Allergy and Infectious Diseases
NIAMD National Institute of Arthritis and Metabolic Diseases
NIB National Institute for the Blind
NIBS Nippon Institute of Biological Sciences
NIBSC National Institute for Biological Standards and Control
NICHHD National Institute of Child Health and Human Development
NICM Nuffield Institute of Comparative Medicine
NICU Neonatal (Newborn) Intensive Care Unit; Neurological Intensive Care Unit
NIDDM noninsulin-dependent diabetes mellitus
NIDM National Institute for Disaster Mobilization
NIDR National Institute of Dental Research
NIEHS National Institute of Environmental Health Services
NIF negative inspiratory force
nig *niger* (L) black
NIGMS National Institute of General Medical Sciences

NIH National Institutes of Health (Bethesda, Md)
NIHL noise-induced hearing loss
NIHR National Institute of Handicapped Research
NIHS National Institute of Hypertension Studies
NIIC National Injury Information Clearinghouse
NIIP National Institute of Industrial Psychology
NIIS National Institute of Infant Services
NIMH National Institute of Mental Health
NIMR National Institute for Medical Research
NINCDS National Institute of Neurological and Communicable Diseases and Stroke
NINDB National Institute of Neurological Diseases and Blindness (NIH)
NIOSH National Institute of Occupational Safety and Health
NIP nipple
NIPH National Institute of Public Health
NIRMP National Intern and Resident Matching Program
NIRNS National Institute for Research in Nuclear Science
NIT National Intelligence Test (psychology)
NIV nodule-inducing virus
NK *Nomenklatur Kommission* (Ger) Commission on Nomenclature
NKH nonketotic hyperglycaemia
nl nanolitre (SI); *non licet* (L) it is not permitted; *non liquet* (L) it is not clear
NLA National Leukemia Association
Nle norleucine
NLEF National Lupus Erythematosus Foundation
NLM National Library of Medicine; noise level monitor
NLN National League for Nursing; no longer needed
NLNE National League for Nursing Education
NLP neurolinguistic programming; no light perception
NLT normal lymphocyte transfer
nlt not less than
NM neuromuscular; nictitating membrane; night and morning; nitrogen mustards; non-motile (with reference to bacteria); non-white male; nuclear medicine
nm nanometre (SI); *nux moschata* (L) nutmeg
NMA National Malaria Association; National Medical Association
NMC National Medical Care; Naval Medical Center
NME National Medical Enterprises, Inc.
NMF National Medical Fellowships; National Migraine

Foundation; non-migrating fraction (of spermatozoa)
NMI no middle initial
NMN nicotinamide mononucleotide
NMNA National Male Nurse Association
NMNRU National Medical Neuropsychiatric Research Unit
NMP Naval Medical Publication
NMR nictitating membrane response; nuclear magnetic resonance (spectroscopy)
NMRDC Naval Medical Research and Development Command
NMRI Naval Medical Research Institute
NMRL Naval Medical Research Laboratory
NMRU Naval Medical Research Unit
NMS Naval Medical School
NMSS National Multiple Sclerosis Society
NMT Nuclear Medicine Technology; neuromuscular tension
NMU neuromuscular unit
N:N the azo group
nn nerves; *nomen novum* (L) new name
NNC National Nutrition Consortium
NND neonatal death; New and Non-official Drugs
NNDC National Naval Dental Center
NNEB National Nursery Examination Board
NNMC National Naval Medical Center
NNN Novy-Nicolle-McNeal (bacteriological culture medium)
n nov *nomen novum* (L) new name
NNP nerve net pulse
NNR New and Non-official Remedies
NO narcotics officer; nitric oxide (chemical formula: N_2O)
no number; *numero* (L) to the number of
NOA National Optometric Association
NOAPP National Organization of Adolescent Pregnancy and Parenting
noct *nocte* (L) at night; *nox, noctis* (L) night, nocturnal
noct maneq *nocte maneque* (L) at night and in the morning
NOEL no observed effect level (of a toxin)
NOF National Osteopathic Foundation
nom dub *nomen dubium* (L) a doubtful name
nom nov *nomen novum* (L) new name
nom nud *nomen nudum* (L) a name without designation

OASP organic acid soluble phosphorus
OB obstetrics; occult bleeding
ob *obiit* (L) he died; she died
OBD organic brain disease
OBE Office of Biological Education; Order of the British Empire; out-of-body experience
OBG obstetrician-gynaecologist
OB-GYN obstetrics-gynaecology
obl oblique
OBS obstetrics; organic brain syndrome
Obs observer, observed; obsolete
Obst obstetrics(-trician)
obst obstruction
OC occlusocervical; office call; only child; oral contraceptive; oxygen consumed
O&C onset and course (of a disease)
Occ occasionally; occlusion
OccTh occupational therapy(-apist)
Occup occupation(al)
OCD Office of Child Development; Office of Civil Defense; ovarian cholesterol depletion (test)
OCN oculomotor nucleus
OCS open canalicular system (of platelets); Outpatient Clinic Substation
OCT ornithine carbonyl transferase; oxytocin challenge test
Octup *octuplus* (L) eight-fold
OCV ordinary conversational voice
OD Doctor of Optometry; occupational disease; *oculus dexter* (L) right eye; open drop; optical density; originally derived; out-of-date; outside diameter; overdose
od *omni die* (L) every day, daily; once daily
ODA *occipito-dextra anterior* (L) right occipitoanterior (position of fetus)
ODB opiate directed behaviour
ODM ophthalmodynamometry
Odont odontology
odoram *odoramentum* (L) a perfume
odorat *odoratus* (L) odorous, smelling, perfuming
ODP *occipito-dextra posterior* (L) right occipitoposterior (position of fetus)
ODT *occipito-dextra transverse* (L) right occipitotransverse (position of fetus)
OE on examination; otitis externa
O&E observation and examination

OEE   outer enamel epithelium

OER   osmotic erythrocyte enrichment; oxygen enhancement ratio

OES   optical emission spectroscopy

oesoph   oesophagus

OF   occipital-frontal (diameter of head); orbitofrontal; osmotic fragility (test)

O/F   oxidation/fermentation (medium)

Off   official

OG   Obstetrics/Gynaecology; occlusogingival; optic ganglion; orange green

OGF   ovarian growth factor

OGM   outgrowth medium

OGTT   oral glucose tolerance test

OH   hydroxyl radical; occupational health; occupational history; *omni hora* (L) every hour; Osteopathic Hospital; Outpatient Hospital

OHC   Occupational Health Center; outer hair cells

OH-Cbl   hydroxycobalamin

OHCS   hydroxycorticosteroid

OHD   hydroxycholecalciferol (activated vitamin D); Office of Human Development (HHS); organic heart disease

OHDA   hydroxydopamine (oxidopamine)

OHI   Occupational Health Institute; ocular hypertension indicator

OHIP   Ontario Health Insurance Plan (Canada)

OHN   Occupational Health Nurse

OHR   Office of Health Research (EPA)

OHS   obesity hypoventilation syndrome

OI   opsonic index; orgasmic impairment; orientation inventory; oxygen income or intake

OID   organism identification number

OIF   Osteogenic Imperfecta Foundation

OIH   ovulation-inducing hormone

oint   ointment

OIP   organizing interstitial pneumonia

OIR   Office of International Research (NIH)

OIT   organic integrity test (psychiatry)

OJ   orange juice

OK   correct, approved, all right

OL   *oculus laevus* (L) left eye

Ol   *oleum* (L) oil

OLA   *occipitolaeva anterior* (L) left occipitoanterior (position of fetus)

oLH   ovine leutenizing hormone

Ol oliv   *oleum olivea* (L) olive oil

OLP   *occipitolaeva posterior* (L) left occipitoposterior (position of fetus)

Ol res   oleoresin

OLT   *occipitolaeva transversa* (L) left occipitotransverse (position of fetus)

OM   occipitomental (diameter of head); Occupational Medicine; Opticalman (Navy); osteomyelitis; otitis media; ovulation method (of birth control)

om   *omni mane* (L) every morning

OMA   Operation Medicare Alert

OME   otitis media with effusion

omn bih   *omni bihora* (L) every two hours

omn hor   *omni hora* (L) every hour

omn 2 hor   *omni secunda hora* (L) every two hours

omn man   *omni mane* (L) every morning

omn noct   *omni nocte* (L) every night

omn quad hor   *omni quadrante hora* (L) every quarter of an hour

OMPA   octamethyl pyrophosphoramide

OM&S   Osteopathic Medicine and Surgery

ON   Office Nurse; optic nerve; Orthopaedic Nurse

on   *omni nocte* (L) every night

ONC   Orthopaedic Nursing Certificate

OND   Ophthalmic Nursing Diploma; other neurological disorders

ONP   operating nursing procedure

ONS   Oncology Nursing Society

ONTG   oral nitroglycerine

ONTR   orders not to resuscitate

OO   oophorectomized

OOB   out of bed; out of body (parapsychology)

OOLR   ophthalmology, otology, laryngology, rhinology

OP   occiput posterior; operation; operative procedure; ophthalmology; osmotic pressure; other than psychotic; outpatient; overproof; ovine prolactin

op   operation; opposite; *opus* (L) work

O&P   ova and parasites

OPC   Outpatient Clinic

OPCA   olivopontocerebellar atrophy

op cit   *opus citatum* (L) in the work cited

OPD   optical path difference; Outpatient Department; Outpatient Dispensary

OpDent   operative dentistry

OPE orbiting primate experiment
opg opening
OPH ophthalmology
Oph ophthalmoscope(-scopic)
OphD Doctor of Ophthalmology
Ophth ophthalmology(-ologic)
OPI oculoparalytic illusion
OPN Ophthalmic Nurse
OPP oxygen partial pressure
opp opposed, opposite
OPS Out-Patient Service
opt optician; optics, optical; optimum; optional
OPV oral poliovirus vaccine
OR oil retention (enema); operating room; orthopaedic; Orthopaedic Research
O-R oxidation-reduction
ORANS Oak Ridge Analytical Systems
Ord orderly
ORDA Office of Recombinant DNA Activities
OREF Orthopedic Research and Education Foundation
org organic
organiz organization(al)
ORIF open reduction with internal fixation
orig origin(al)
OrJ orange juice
ORL otorhinolaryngology
ORN Operating Room Nurse; Orthopaedic Nurse
Orn ornithine
ORNL Oak Ridge National Laboratory
ORO Orapouche (an arbovirus)
ORP oxidation-reduction potential
ORS oral surgeon; Orthopaedic Research Society; orthopaedic surgeon(ery)
ORT operating room technician; oral rehydration therapy
Ortho orthopaedics
OS occupational safety; *oculus sinister* (L) left eye; opening snaps (cardiology); Orthopaedic Surgery; Osgood-Schlatter's (disease); osteogenic sarcoma; osteosarcoma
Os bone (L); mouth (L); osmium
OSA Office of Services to the Aging; Optical Society of America
OSF outer spiral fibres (of the cochlea)
OSH Occupational Safety and Health

OSHA Occupational Safety and Health Act

Osm osmole

osm osmotic

OSRD Office of Scientific Research and Development (USA)

OSS Office of Space Science; Office of Strategic Services (US)

OST Office of Science and Technology

Osteo osteomyelitis; osteopath(y)

OStJ Officer of the Order of St John of Jerusalem

OSTS Office of State Technical Services

OSUK Ophthalmological Society of the United Kingdom

OT objective test (psychology); occupational therapy (-apist); old term; old tuberculin; olfactory threshold; orotracheal; otology

Ot otolaryngology(-ologist)

OTA Office of Technology Assessment; orthotoluidine arsenite (test for blood in urine)

OTC ornithine transcarbamylase; over-the-counter (with reference to drugs not requiring a prescription); oxytetracycline

OTD organ tolerance dose; oral temperature device

OTF oral transfer factor

OTM orthotoluidine manganese sulphate

OTO otology

Otol otology(-ologist)

OTR ovarian tumour registry; Registered Occupational Therapist

OTReg Occupational Therapist Registered (Canada)

OU *oculi unitas* (L) both eyes together; *oculus uterque* (L) for each eye

OV office visit; ovalbumin; overventilation (hyperventilation); ovulating (women)

ov *ovum* (L) egg

OVD occlusal vertical dimension

OVLT organum vasculosum of the lamina terminalis

OVRR Office of Vocational Rehabilitation

OVX ovariectomized

OW ordinary welfare; out-of-wedlock

O/W oil in water (with reference to emulsions)

OWA organics-in-water analyser

OX oxacillin

ox oxymel (honey, water, and vinegar)

OXY oxygen; oxytocin

oz ounce

P

P page; pain; *parte* (L) part; partial pressure or tension; *Pasteurella; pater* (L) father; paternally contributing; patient; *per* (L) by; percentile; perceptual speed; percussion; perforation; peyote; pharmacopoeia; phenylalanine; phenolphthalein; phosphate; phosphorus; physiology; pink; plasma; placebo; pole; *pondere* (L) by weight; poise (unit of dynamic viscosity); poison; polymyxin; population; porcelain; porphyrin; position; positive; posterior; postpartum; prednisone; premolar; presbyopia; President; pressure; primary; primitive (with reference to haemoglobin); probability; product; prolactin; proprionic; *proximum* (L) near; psychiatry (-iatrist); *pugillus* (L) handful; pulse; *punctum proximum* (L) near point (of vision); pupil

p page; papilla (optic); pico (prefix) (SI); pint; *post* (L) after; pupil

π pi

p- *para-* (in chemical formulas)

P₁ first parental generation (in genetics)

P₂ second pulmonic heart sound

³²P radioactive phosphorus

PA Paleopathology Association; paralysis agitans; paranoia; pernicious anaemia; phosphatidic acid; phosphoarginine; photoallergic (response); Physician's Assistant; pituitary-adrenal; plasma aldosterone; plasminogen activator; platelet adhesiveness; polyarteritis; posteroanterior; prealbumin; prior to admission; proactivator; prolonged action; proprietary association; psychoanalyst; psychogenic aspermia; pulmonary artery; pulmonary atresia; pulpo-axial; pyrrolizidine alkaloid

Pₐ partial pressure in arterial blood

Pa Pascal (SI)

P&A percussion and auscultation

PAA phenylacetic acid; pyridineacetic acid

PAB *para*-aminobenzoic (acid); purple agar base medium

PABA *para*-aminobenzoic acid

PAC parent-adult-child (in transactional analysis); phenacetin (acetophenetidin), aspirin, caffeine; premature atrial contraction

PACC protein A immobilized in collodion charcoal

PACE personalized aerobics for cardiovascular enhancement

PaCO₂ arterial carbon dioxide tension

PAD phenacetin, aspirin, desoxyephedrine (methylamphetamine); pulsatile assist device

pae *partes aequales* (L) in equal parts

paed paediatrics

PAF platelet aggregation factor; pseudoamniotic fluid; pulmonary arteriovenous fistula

PA&F percussion, auscultation, and fremitus

PAG pariaqueductal grey matter; polyacrylamide gel electrophoresis

PAH *para*-aminohippuric acid; pulmonary artery hypotension

PAHO Pan-American Health Organization

PAIgG platelet-associated immunoglobulin G

PAL Pathology Laboratory (test); posterior axillary line

palp palpable

palpi palpitation

PAM crystalline penicillin G in 2% aluminium monostearate; primary amoebic meningoencephalitis; pulmonary alveolar macrophages

pam pamphlet

PAN polyarteritis nodosa; positional alcohol nystagmus

PAO peak acid output

PAo pulmonary artery occlusion pressure (wedge pressure)

PaO₂ arterial partial pressure of oxygen

PAP peak airway pressure; peroxidase antiperoxidase; primary atypical pneumonia; prostatic acid phosphatase

Pap Papanicolaou (diagnosis, smear, stain, or test)

pap papilla(e)

PAPP pregnancy associated plasma protein

PAPUFA physiologically active polyunsaturated fatty acids

PAR photosynthetically active radiation; physiological aging rate; postanaesthetic recovery (room); probable allergic rhinitis; Program for Alcohol Recovery

par paraffin

Para Formula designating: P—number of pregnancies; a—number of abortions or miscarriages; ra—number of living children (e.g. Para 4–2–1 means 4 pregnancies, 2 abortions or miscarriages, 1 living child)

Para I unipara (having borne one child)

Para II bipara (having borne two children)

Para III tripara (having borne three children)
par aff *pars affecta* (L) to the part affected
Parapsych parapsychology
Parasit parasitology
parasym div parasympathetic division (of autonomic nervous system)
PARC Palo Alto Research Center
parent parenteral(ly)
parox paroxysmal
part *partim* (L) part
part aeq *partes aequales* (L) in equal parts
part dolent *partes dolentes* (L) painful parts
part vic *partibus vicibus* (L) in divided doses
PARU postanaesthetic recovery unit
parv *parvus* (L) small
PAS *para*-aminosalicylic acid; periodic-acid-Schiff (stain); Professional Activities Study (Commission on Professional and Hospital Activities); progressive accumulated stress
PASA *para*-aminosalicylic acid
P'ase alkaline phosphatase
PASM periodic acid-silver methenamine
pass passive
Past *Pasteurella*
PAT paroxysmal atrial tachycardia; patient; pregnancy at term; psychoacoustic testing
pat patent(ed)
PATE Psychodynamic and Therapeutic Education
PATH pituitary adrenocorticotrophic hormone
Path pathogenic; pathological; pathology(-ologist)
pat med patent medicine
PAWP pulmonary arterial wedge pressure
PB phenobarbitone; phonetically balanced (with reference to word lists); pressure breathing
Pb *plumbum* (L) lead; presbyopia
PBA phenylboronate agarose; polyclonal B-cell activities; Pressure Breathing Assister
PBB polybromated biphenyls
PBBH Peter Bent Brigham Hospital (Boston)
PBC peripheral blood cells; point of basal convergence; primary biliary cirrhosis
PBE *Persucht Bacillen-Emulsion* (Ger) (a form of tuberculin)
PBG porphobilinogen
PBI phenformin; protein-bound iodine

PBK phosphorylase b kinase
PBL peripheral blood leucocyte
PBM peripheral blood mononuclear (cells)
PBME Physiology and Biomedical Engineering (Program)
PBP penicillin-binding protein
PBPE Population Biology/Physiological Ecology
PBS phosphate buffered saline
PBV pulmonary blood volume
PBW posterior bite wing (dentistry)
PBZ phenylbutazone; pyribenzamine (tripelennamine)
PC packed cells; parent cells; Pharmacy Corps; phosphatidylcholine (lecithin); phosphocreatine; phosphorylcholine; Physicians Corporation; plasmacytoma; platelet concentrate; pneumotaxic centre; *pondus civile* (L) avoirdupois weight; postcoital; praecordium; precaution category; present complaint; Prosthetics Center; pseudoconditioning control; pubococcygeus (muscle); pulmonary capillary; pure clairvoyance
pc per cent; picocurie; *post cibos* (L) after meals; *post cibum* (L) after food
PCA passive cutaneous anaphylaxis; President's Council on Aging; procoagulant activity
PCB polychlorinated biphenyls; procarbazine
PcB near point of convergence to the intercentral base line
PCC phaeochromocytoma; phosphate carrier compound; Poison Control Center; premature chromosome condensation; prothrombin-complex concentration
PCc periscopic concave
PCD plasma cell dyscrasia; polycystic disease; pulmonary clearance delay
PCDUS plasma cell dyscrasia of unknown significance
PCE pseudocholinesterase; pulmocutaneous exchange
PCF pharyngoconjunctival fever; prothrombin conversion factor
PCG paracervical ganglion; phonocardiogram; pubococcygeus (muscle)
PCH paroxysmal cold haemoglobinuria
pCi picocurie (SI)
PCIC Poison Control Information Center
PCKD polycystic kidney disease
PCL persistent corpus luteum; posterior cruciate ligament

PCM protein-calorie malnutrition; protein-carboxyl methylase

PCMO Principal Clinical Medical Officer (Brit); Principal Colonial Medical Officer

PCMU physico-chemical measurements unit (Brit)

PCN penicillin; pregnenolone carbonitril; Primary Care Nursing

PCNV Provisional Committee on Nomenclature of Viruses

PCO patient complains of; polycystic ovary

PCOB Permanent Central Opium Board (Geneva)

PCO₂ carbon dioxide pressure or tension

PCP Patient Care Publications; pentachlorophenol; pneumocystic pneumonia; Primary Care Physician

PCPA p-chlorophenylalanine (fenclonine)

pcpn precipitation

pcpt perception

PCS palliative care service; Patterns of Care Study; primary cancer site

pcs preconscious

PCSM percutaneous stone manipulation

PCT plasmacrit test (syphilis); plasmacytoma; porphyria cutanea tarda; proximal convoluted tubule (of a nephron)

pct per cent

PCU Pain Control Unit

PCV packed cell volume; polycythaemia vera; porcine cirovirus

PCW primary capillary wedge

PD Doctor of Pharmacy; Dublin Pharmacopoeia; interpupillary distance; paediatrics; paralysing dose; parkinsonism dementia; Parkinson's disease; pars distalis (pituitary); peritoneal dialysis; phenyldichlorarsine; phosphate dextrose (media); poorly differentiated; postnasal drainage; potential difference; pressor dose; psychopathic deviate; psychotic depression; pulpodistal

pd papilla diameter; *per diem* (L) by the day; prism diopter; pupillary distance

PDA paediatric allergy; patent ductus arteriosus

PDB paradichlorobenzene; phosphorus-dissolving bacteria

PDC paediatrics-cardiology; penta-decylcatechol; preliminary diagnostic clinic; private diagnostic clinic

PDE paroxysmal dyspnoea on exertion; phosphodiesterase

PDF Parkinson's Disease Foundation
PDGA pteroyldiglutamic acid
PDGF platelet-derived growth factor
PDH past dental history
PDHC pyruvate dehydrogenase complex
PDI Psychomotor Development Index
P-diol pregnanediol
PDLL poorly differentiated lymphocytic lymphoma
PDQ at once; immediately
PDR paediatrics-radiology; Physicians' Desk Reference; proliferative diabetic retinopathy
pdr powder
PdS psychiatric deviate, subtile
PDUR Predischarge Utilization Review (Program)
PE Edinburgh Pharmacopoeia; pharyngo-esophageal; physical examination; physical exercise; Physiological Ecology; potential energy; powdered extract; practical exercise; probable error; pulmonary embolism
Pe pressure on expiration
PEA phenethyl alcohol (blood agar)
PEC peritoneal exudate cells; pyogenic exotoxin C
PED pediatrics
PEd physical education
PEDG phenformin
PeDS Pediatric Drug Surveillance (Program)
PEEP positive end expiratory pressure
PEF peak expiratory flow; Psychiatric Evaluation Form
PEFV partial expiratory flow-volume
PEG pneumoencephalography(-ogram); polyethylene glycol
PEI phosphorus excretion index
PEL peritoneal exudate lymphocytes
PEM prescription-event monitoring; primary enrichment medium; probable error of measurement
PEMS Physical, Emotional, Mental Safety
Pen penicillin
penic penicillin
penic cam *penicillum camelinum* (L) camel's-hair brush
PEN-O Penner serotype-O
Pent pentothal (thiopentone sodium)
PEP phosphoenolpyruvate; physiological evaluation of primates; polyestradiol phosphate; pre-ejection period
PEPI pre-ejection period index
PER protein efficiency ratio
Per permission

per by; through; period; periodic; person
perf perforation(-ated)
periap periapical
PERLA pupils equal, react to light and accommodation
perm permanent
per op emet *peracta operatione emetici* (L) when the action of emetic is over
perp perpendicular
PERRLA pupils equal, round, react to light and accommodation
pers personal
pert pertussis (whooping cough)
PES Physicians Equity Services; pre-excitation syndrome
PESS *pessus* (L) pessary
PET pre-eclamptic toxaemia; positron emission tomography; Psychiatry Emergency Team
PETN pentaerythritol tetraniconitate (niceritrol); pentaerythritol tetranitrate
petr petroleum
PF peak flow; permeability factor; phenylalanine and methotrexate; plantar flexion; platelet factor; protection factor; pulmonary factor
Pf *Pfeifferella*
PFA *para*-fluorophenylalanine
PFC perfluorocarbons; plaque-forming cells
PFD primary flash distillate
PFK phosphofructokinase
PFO patent foramen ovale
PFP platelet-free plasma
PFR peak flow rate (reading)
PFS pulmonary function score
PFT pancreatic function test; phenylalanine mustard (melphalan), fluorouracil, tamoxifen; pulmonary function test
PFU plaque-forming unit; pock-forming units
PFV physiological full value
PG glycerate-3-phosphate; *paralysie générale* (Fr) general paralysis; paregoric; Pharmacopoeia Germanica; phosphatidylglycerol; phosphogluconate; plasma glucose; postgraduate; pregnanediol glucuronide; prostaglandin
Pg pregnant
pg picogram (SI)
PGA prostaglandin A; pteroylglutamic acid (folic acid)
PGB prostaglandin B

PGC   primordial germ cell
PGD   prostaglandin D
PGDF Pilot Guide Dog Foundation
PGE   prostaglandin E
PGF   prostaglandin F
PGFM prostaglandin F and its metabolite (dihydro-keto-
          prostaglandin)
PGH   pituitary growth hormone; prostaglandin H
PGI$_2$ prostacyclin
PGL   phosphoglycolipid
PGM   phosphoglucomutase
PGN   proliferative glomerulonephritis
PGR   psychogalvanic response
PgR   progesterone receptor
PGS   plant growth substance
PGU   postgonococcal urethritis
PGUT phosphogalactose-uridyl transferase
PGYE peptone, glucose yeast extract (medium)
PH   past history; porta hepatis; previous history; public
          health
Ph   pharmacopoeia; phenyl; phosphate
pH   Symbol for expression of hydrogen ion concentration
ph   phial
PHA   passive haemagglutination; peripheral hyperali-
          mentation solution; phytohaemagglutinin
phaeo phaeochromocytoma
phar(m) pharmacopoeia; pharmaceutical; pharmacy
PharB *Pharmaciae Baccalaureus* (L) Bachelor of
          Pharmacy
PharC Pharmaceutical Chemist
PharD *Pharmaciae Doctor* (L) Doctor of Pharmacy
PharG Graduate in Pharmacy
PHARM pharmacy, pharmacist
PharM *Pharmaciae Magister* (L) Master of Pharmacy
PHB   Public Health Bibliography
PhB   Bachelor of Philosophy
PHC   posthospital care; premolar aplasia, hyperhydrosis,
          and premature canities; primary hepatic carcinoma;
          proliferative helper cells
PhC   Pharmaceutical Chemist
Ph^{1}c Philadelphia chromosome
PhD   Doctor of Pharmacy; Doctor of Philosophy
PHE   post-heparin esterase
Phe   phenylalanine
Pheo phaeochromocytoma

PHF   Personal Hygiene Facility
PHFG   primary human fetal glia
PhG   Graduate in Pharmacy; Pharmacopoeia Germanica
Phgly   phenylglycine
PHI   phosphohexose isomerase; physiological hyaluronidase inhibitor
PhI   Pharmacopoeia Internationalis
phial   *phiala* (L) bottle
PHIM   posthypoxic intention myoclonus
PHIS   Physically Handicapped in Science
PHK   postmorten human kidney (cells)
PHL   Public Health Law
PHLA   post-heparin lipolytic activity
PHLS   Public Health Laboratory Service (Brit)
PHLSB   Public Health Laboratory Service Board
PHM   Pharmacist's Mate (Navy)
PhM   Master in Pharmacy
PHMDP   Pharmacist's Mate, Dental Prosthetic Technician (Navy)
PhmG   Graduate in Pharmacy
PHN   Public Health Nursing
phos   phosphate; phosphorus
PHP   post-heparin phospholipase; prepaid health plan; pseudohypoparathyroidism
PHR   peak heart rate; Public Health Reports
PHS   posthypnotic suggestion; Public Health Service
PHSP   Public Health Service Publications
PhTD   Physical Therapy Doctor
PHTS   Psychiatric Home Treatment Service
PHY   pharyngitis; physical
PHYS   physiology(-ological)
PhyS   physiological saline
Phys   physician
phys   physical
phys dis   physical disability
PhysEd   physical education
physio   physiotherapy(-apist)
Physiol   physiology(-ological)
PhysMed   physical medicine
PhysTher   physical therapy
PI   patient's interests; perinatal injury; personal injury; personality inventory; Pharmacopoeia Internationalis; physically impaired; pneumatosis intestinalis; poison ivy; pregnancy induced; present illness; primary infarction; proactive inhibition (psychology); prolactin

inhibitor; protamine insulin; protean inhibitor; Protocol Internationale (International Protocol); Psychiatric Institute; pulmonary incompetence

Pi pressure of inspiration

PIA Psychiatric Institute of America

PIC postinflammatory corticoid

PICU Paediatric Intensive Care Unit; Pulmonary Intensive Care Unit

PID pelvic inflammatory disease; photoionization detector; prolapsed inververtebral disc

PIDRA portable insulin dosage-regulating apparatus

PIE preimplantation embryo; pulmonary infiltration associated with eosinophilia

PIF prolactin release inhibiting factor; proliferation inhibiting factor

PIFR peak inspiratory flow rate

PIFT platelet immunofluorescence test

pigm *pigmentum* (L) paint

PIH pregnancy induced hypertension; prolactin-release inhibiting hormone

PII primary irritation indices

pil *pilula* (L) pill

PIMCO Physicians Insurance Medical Company

ping *pinguis* (L) fat, grease

PIP piperacillin; proximal interphalangeal (joint)

PIR postinhibitory rebound

PIRP Provisional International Reference Preparation

PIS Provisional International Standard

PIT picture identification test

PITR plasma iron turnover rate

PIV parainfluenza virus

PK Prausnitz-Küstner (reaction); psychokinesis; pyruvate kinase

pK dissociation constant

PKase protein kinase

PKU phenylketonuria

PL palm leaf reaction; perception of light; phospholipid; photoluminescence; placebo; placental lactogen; plastic surgeon (surgery); pulpolingual

pl place; plate; plural

PLA phospholipase A; pulpolinguoaxial

PLa pulpolabial

plant-flex plantar flexion

PLB phospholipase B

PLC proinsulin-like compound

PLD potentially lethal damage
PLG plasminogen
P-LGV psittacosis-lymphogranuloma venereum
PLL peripheral light loss
PLM polarized light microscopy
PLN posterior lip nerve
PLP pyridoxal phosphate
PLT platelet; psittacosis-lymphogranuloma venereum-trachoma
plumb *plumbum* (L) lead
plx plexus
PM pacemaker; *petit mal;* physical medicine; poliomyelitis; polymorphs; polymyositis; *post meridiem* (L) after noon; *post mortem* (L) after death; premolar; presystolic murmur; preventive medicine; prostatic massage; pulpomesial
PMA papillary, marginal, attached (with reference to gingivae); Pharmaceutical Manufacturers Association; phosphomolybdic acid; Primary Mental Abilities (test); progressive muscular atrophy; pyridylmercuric acetate
PMB polychrome methylene blue; polymorphonuclear basophils; post-menopausal bleeding
PMC Pacific Medical Center; phenylmercuric chloride; pseudomembranous colitis
PMD primary myocardial disease; progressive muscular dystrophy
PMd private physician
PME polymorphonuclear eosinophils
PMF progressive massive fibrosis
PMH past medical history
PMI past (previous) medical illness; patient medication instruction; point of maximal impulse (of heart on chest wall); point of maximum intensity; present medical illness
PML polymorphonuclear leucocytes; posterior mitral leaflet; progressive multifocal leucoencephalopathy
PMN polymorphonuclear; polymorphonuclear neutrophils
PMNL polymorphonuclear leucocyte
PMNR periadenitis mucosa necrotica recurrens
PMO postmenopausal osteoporosis; Principal Medical Officer
PMP persistent mentoposterior (position of fetus); previous menstrual period
PMQ phytlylmenaquinone (vitamin K)

PMR physical medicine and rehabilitation; polymyalgia rheumatica; proportionate mortality ratio; protein magnetic resonance

PM&R physical medicine and rehabilitation

PMRAFNS Princess Mary's Royal Air Force Nursing Service

PMRS Physical Medicine and Rehabilitation Service

PMS chorionic gonadotrophin in pregnant mare's serum; poor miserable soul; post-menopausal syndrome; pregnant mare's serum; premenstrual syndrome

PMSG pregnant mare's serum gonadotrophin

PMT premenstrual tension

PN percussion note; periarteritis nodosa; peripheral nerve; polyarteritis nodosa; postnatal; Practical Nurse; psychiatry-neurology; psycho-neurologist; psycho-neurotic individual

Pn pneumonia

P&N psychiatry and neurology

PNA Nomina Anatomica (Paris) (with reference to anatomical nomenclature); pentosenucleic acid

PNAvQ positive-negative ambivalent quotient (psychology)

PNBT *para*-nitro blue tetrazolium

PNC penicillin; pneumotaxic centre; pseudonurse cells

PND paroxysmal nocturnal dyspnoea; postnasal drip or drainage

PNE Practical Nurse's Education

PNed *Nederlandsche Pharmacopee* (Dutch pharmacopoeia)

PNF proprioceptive neuromuscular facilitation

PNH paroxysmal nocturnal haemoglobinuria

PNI peripheral nerve injury; postnatal infection

PNK polynucleotide kinase

PNMT phenylethanolamine-N-methyl transferase

PNO Principal Nursing Officer

PNP peripheral neuropathy; purine nucleotide phosphorylase

P-NP *p*-nitrophenol

PNPR positive-negative pressure respiration

PNS parasympathetic nervous system; peripheral nervous system

PNT patient

PNU protein nitrogen unit

Pnx pneumothorax

PO period of onset; phone order; postoperative

po *per os* (L) by mouth
PO₂ oxygen tension or pressure
PO₄ phosphate
POA pancreatic oncofetal antigen; phalangeal osteoarthritis; preoptic area; primary optic atrophy
POB penicillin, oil beeswax
POC purgeable organic carbon
pocill *pocillum* (L) a small cup
pocul *poculum* (L) cup
POD peroxidase
PODx preoperative diagnosis
POE postoperative endophthalmitis
POF pyruvate oxidation factor
PofE portal of entry
pOH Symbol used in expressing hydroxyl (OH) concentration, or alkalinity, of a solution
POHI physically or otherwise health-impaired
POI Personal Orientation Inventory
pois poison
pol polish (dentistry)
polio poliomyelitis
POLL *pollex* (L) inch
Poly polymorphonuclear leucocyte or neutrophil granulocyte
POMC propriomelanocortin
POMR problem oriented medical record
PON particulate organic nitrogen
pond *pondere* (L) by weight
POP paroxypropione; persistent occipitoposterior (position of fetus); plasma osmotic pressure; plaster of paris
POp postoperative
Pop popliteal; population
pop popular
POS polycystic ovarian syndrome
pos position; positive
POSM patient-operated selector mechanism
POSS proximal over-shoulder strap
post posterior; postmortem (autopsy)
postgangl postganglionic
post-op postoperative
POT *potus* (L) a drink
pot potassium; potential; potion
potass potassium
POU placenta, ovary, uterus
POW Powassan encephalitis

powd powder
PP pancreatic polypeptide; partial pressure; placental protein; Planned Parenthood; plasma protein; Population Planning; posterior pituitary; postpartum; post-prandial; private patient; private practice; pulse pressure; pyrophosphate
pp *punctum proximum* (L) near point of accommodation (in respect to vision)
PPA phenylpropanolamine; Pittsburgh pneumonia agent; Population Planning Associates; post-partum amenorrhoea
ppa *phiala prius agitate* (L) the bottle having first been shaken
pp&a palpation, percussion, and auscultation
PPB positive pressure breathing
ppb parts per billion
PPC progressive patient care; proximal palmar crease
PPCA plasma prothrombin conversion accelerator
PPCF plasma prothrombin conversion factor
PPD progressive perceptive deafness; purified protein derivative (tuberculin)
PPD-S purified protein derivative-standard
PPE porcine pancreatic elastase
PPF pellagra preventive factor (niacinamide); plasma protein fraction
PPFA Planned Parenthood Federation of America
ppg picopicogram
PPGF polypeptide growth factor
PPH post-partum haemorrhage
PPHP pseudo-pseudohypoparathyroidism
PPI patient package insert
PPLO pleuropneumonia-like organisms
PPM phosphopentomutase
ppm parts per million
PPNA peak phrenic nerve activity
PPO platelet peroxidase; pleuropneumonia organisms; preferred-provider organization
PPP platelet-poor plasma; polyphoretic phosphate
PPRWP poor precordial R-wave progression
PPS Personal Preference Scale; post-partum sterilization
PPSB prothrombin, proconvertin, Stuart factor, anti-haemophilic B factor
PPT partial prothrombin time
ppt precipitate; prepared
pptd precipitated

PPTL postpartum tubal ligation
pptn precipitation
PQ permeability quotient
PR Panama red (type of marijuana); parallax and refraction; partial remission; partial response; patient relations; percentile rank; peripheral resistance; per rectum; phenol red; pityriasis rosea; pregnancy rate; pressoreceptor; pressure; prevention; proctologist; progesterone receptor; progressive resistance; prolactin; prosthetic-group removing (enzyme); prosthion; pulse rate
Pr presbyopia; presentation; prism; prolactin; propyl
pr pair; per rectum; *punctum remotum* (L) far point of accommodation (in respect to vision)
PRA plasma renin activity
prac practice
PRACT practitioner
pract practical
prand *prandium* (L) dinner
PRAS prereduced anaerobically sterilized (media)
p rat aetat *pro ratione aetatis* (L) in proportion to age
PRB Personnel Reaction Blank; Prosthetics Research Board
PRC plasma renin concentration
PRCA pure red cell aplasia
PRD partial reaction of degeneration
PRE photoreactivity; progressive resistive exercise
Pre preliminary
p rec per rectum
precip precipitate(-ation)
PRED prednisone
PreD$_3$ previtamin D$_3$
pred predicted
prefd preferred
preg pregnant
pregang preganglionic
pregn pregnant
prelim preliminary
prelim diag preliminary diagnosis
prem premature; premature infant
premie premature infant
pre-op preoperative
prep prepare(-ation)
prepd prepared
prepn preparation

preserv preserve(-ation)
press pressure
prev prevent(ion)(ative); previous
PrevMed preventative medicine
PREVMEDU Preventative Medicine Unit
pre-voc pre-vocational
PRF partial reinforcement; pontine reticular formation; prolactin-releasing factor
PRG purge
PRH prolactin-releasing hormone
PRIH prolactin-release inhibiting hormone
prim luc *prima luc* (L) early in the morning
prim m *primo mane* (L) early in the morning
prin principal
PRIST paper radioimmunosorbent test
priv private
PRL prolactin
PRM photoreceptor membrane
prn *pro re nata* (L) as required, whenever necessary
PRO pronation
Pro proline; prophylactic; prothrombin
prob probability; probable(-ly); problem
proc procedure; proceeding; process
Procs proceedings
Proct proctology(-ologist)
prod product
Prof professor
prof profession(al)
prog prognosis; program; progressive
progn prognosis
progr progress
proj project
prolong *prolongatus* (L) prolonged
PROM premature rupture of membranes
pron pronation
proph prophylactic
pro rect *pro recto* (L) by rectum
pros prostate
prosth prosthesis
Prot Protestant
prot protein
pro-time prothrombin time
PROTO protoporphyrin
PROVIMI proteins, vitamins, and minerals
prox proximal

PRO-XAN protein-xanthophyll

prox luc *proxima luce* (L) the day before

PRP platelet-rich plasma; pressure rate product; progressive rubella panencephalitis; Psychotic Reaction Profile

PRPP phosphoribosyl pyrophosphate

PR-RSV Prague strain Rous sarcoma virus

PRS Personality Rating Scale

PRT pharmaceutical research and testing; phosphoribosyl transferase

PRU peripheral resistance unit

PRV pseudorabies virus

PS chloropicrin; paediatric surgery; paradoxical sleep; pathological stage; patient's serum; perceptial speed (test); phosphate saline (buffer); phosphatidyl serine; photosystems; physical status; plastic surgery; point of symmetry; postscriptum; pulmonary stenosis; serum from a pregnant woman

P/S polyunsaturated/saturated (fatty acid ratio)

Ps prescription (with reference to drugs requiring a prescription); *Pseudomonas*

ps pseudo

P&S paracentesis and suction (with reference to thoracic surgery); Physicians and Surgeons

PSA prolonged sleep apnea; prostate specific antigen

PSAn psychoanalyst(-analysis)(-analytic)(-analytical)

PSB phosphorus-solubilizing bacteria; protected specimen brush

PSC primary sclerosing cholangitis; pulse synchronized contractions

PSF pseudosarcomatous fasciitis

PSG phosphate-saline-glucose buffer

PSGN poststreptococcal glomerulonephritis

PSI posterior sagittal index; Problem Solving Information (apparatus); psychosomatic inventory

psi pounds per square inch

psai pounds per square inch absolute

psig pounds per square inch gauge

PSIL preferred-frequency speech interference level

PSL sol potassium, sodium chloride, sodium lactate solution

PSMA progressive spinal muscular atrophy

PSMed Psychosomatic Medicine

P sol partly soluble

PSP pace-setting potential; parathyroid secretory protein; phenolsulphonphthalein (phenol red); pseudopregnancy

psp postsynaptic potential

PSR pain sensitivity range; pulmonary stretch receptors

PSRC Plastic Surgery Research Council

PSRO Professional Standards Review Organization

PSS physiological saline solution; progressive systemic sclerosis; Psychiatric Services Section (American Hospital Association)

PST penicillin, streptomycin and tetracycline; poststimulus time

PSurg plastic surgery

PSV psychological, social and vocational (adjustment factors)

PSVT paroxysmal supraventricular tachycardia

PSW Psychiatric Social Worker

PSWT Psychiatric Social Work Training (Brit)

Psy psychiatry

psych psychology

PSYCHEM psychiatric chemistry

psychiat psychiatry(-iatric)

psychoan psychoanalysis

psychol psychology

psychopathol psychopathology(-ological)

psychophys psychophysics

psychophysiol psychophysiology

PsychosMed Psychosomatic Medicine

psychother psychotherapy

psy-path psychopath(ic)

psy-som psychosomatic

PT parathyroid; patient; phototoxicity; physical therapy; physical training; physiotherapy; polyvalent tolerance; propylthiouracil; prothrombin time; pulmonary tuberculosis; pyramidal tract

Pt platinum

pt part; patient; *perstetur* (L) let it be continued; pint; point

PTA percutaneous transluminal angioplasty; plasma thromboplastin antecedent (Factor XI); post-traumatic amnesia; prior to admission

PTAP purified toxoid (diphtheria) precipitated by aluminium phosphate

p'tase phosphatase

PTB patellar tendon bearing; prior to birth

PTC percutaneous transhepatic cholangiogram; phenylthiocarbamide (phenylthiourea); plasma thromboplastin component (Factor IX, Christmas factor); posterior trabeculae carnea; prothrombin complex

PTCA percutaneous transluminal coronary angioplasty
PTD permanent total disability
PTE parathyroid extract
PteGlu pteroylglutamic acid (folic acid)
PTF plasma thromboplastin factor (Factor X)
PTH parathormone (parathyroid hormone); post-transfusion hepatitis
PTI persistent tolerant infection
PTL perinatal telencephalic leucoencephalopathy
PTLD prescribed tumour lethal dose
PTM post-transfusion mononucleosis; preterm milk
PTO *Perlsucht-Tuberculin Original* (Ger) (Spengler's tuberculin)
PTP post-tetanic potentiation
Ptp transpulmonary pressure
PTR *Perlsucht-Tuberculin Rest* (Ger)
PTSD post-traumatic stress disorder
PTT partial thromboplastin time; pulmonary transit time
PTTH prothoracicotropic hormone
PTU propylthiouracil
PTx parathyroidectomy
PTXA parathyroidectomy and autotransplantation
PU passed urine; peptic ulcer; per urethra; pregnancy urine
Pu plutonium; purple
pub public; publisher(-shed)
PuD pulmonary disease
PUFA polyunsaturated fatty acid
PUH pregnancy urine hormone
PUL pulmonary
pulm *pulmentum* (L) gruel; pulmonary
pulv *pulvis* (L) powder
pulv gros *pulvis grossus* (L) a coarse powder
pulv subtil *pulvis subtilis* (L) a smooth powder
pulv tenu *pulvis tenuis* (L) an extremely fine powder
PUO pyrexia of unknown origin
PUR polyurethane
purg *purgativus* (L) cathartic, purgative
PUVA psoralens and ultraviolet A (therapy)
PV paraventricular (nucleus); paromomycin-vancomycin blood agar; per vaginam; plasma volume; polycythaemia vera; polyoma virus; portal vein; pressure/volume; pulmonary vein

PVA   polyvinyl alcohol (fixative)
PVB   premature ventricular beat
PVBS   possible vertebral-basilar system
PVC   polyvinylchloride; premature ventricular contraction; primary visual cortex
PVD   peripheral vascular disease; pulmonary vascular disease
PVF   peripheral visual field
PVH   preventricular haemorrhage
PVI   peripheral vascular insufficiency; personal values inventory
P-VL   Panton-Valentine leucocidin
PVM   pneumonia virus of mice; proteins, vitamins, minerals
PVMed   Preventative Medicine
PVNPS   Post-Viet Nam Psychiatric Syndrome
PVOD   peripheral vascular occlusive disease
PVP   polyvinylpyrrolidone (povidone)
PVP-I   povidone-iodine
PVR   pulmonary vascular resistance; pulse volume recording
PVS   persistent vegetative state; plexus visibility score
PVT   paroxysmal ventricular tachycardia; pressure, volume, temperature; private patient
pvt   private
PW   psychological warfare
Pw   progesterone withdrawal
PWBC   peripheral white blood cells
PWC   peak work capacity; physical working capacity
PWM   pokeweed mitogen
PWP   pulmonary wedge pressure
PX   pancreatectomized; physical examination
Px   past history; pneumothorax; prognosis
PXE   pseudoxanthoma elasticum
PXM   projection X-ray microscope
Py   phosphopyridoxal
PYA   psychoanalysis
PYC   proteose-yeast, castione (medium)
PyC   pyogenic culture
PYE   peptone yeast extract (medium)
PYG   peptone yeast extract glucose (medium)
PYGM   peptone-yeast glucose maltose (agar/broth)
PYM   psychosomatic medicine
Pyr   pyridine; pyruvate
PyrP   pyridoxyl (pyridoxamine) phosphate

PZ pancreozymin
PZA pyrazinamide
PZI protamine zinc insulin
PZP pregnancy zone protein

Q

Q quantity; quartile; query or Queensland (fever); quinacrine (fluorescent method); quinone; quotient; volume of blood
Q_1, Q_2, Q_3 first or lowest quartile, second quartile, third quartile
q *quaque* (L) each, every
QAC quaternary ammonium compound
qam every morning
QAP quality assurance program; quinine, atabrine, plasmoquinum (pamaquin) (treatment)
QARANC Queen Alexandra's Royal Army Nursing Corps
QARNNS Queen Alexandra's Royal Naval Nursing Service
QCH Queen Charlotte's Hospital
QCIM Quarterly Cumulative Index Medicus
qd *quaque die* (L) every day
qds *quater die sumendum* (L) to be taken four times a day
QEH Queen Elizabeth's Hospital
QEONS Queen Elizabeth's Overseas Nursery Service
QEW quick early warning (test)
QF quick freeze
Q fract quick fraction (with reference to membrane potentials)
qh *quaque hora* (L) every hour
q2h *quaque secunda hora* (L) every two hours
q3h *quaque tertia hora* (L) every three hours
QHDS Queen's Honorary Dental Surgeon
QHNS Queen's Honorary Nursing Sister
QHP Honorary Physician to the Queen
QHS Honorary Surgeon to the Queen
qid *quater in die* (L) four times a day
QIDN Queen's Institute of District Nursing
ql *quantum libet* (L) as much as is desired, as much as you please

qm *quaque mane* (L) every morning
qn *quaque nocte* (L) once every night
QNS quantity not sufficient; Queen's Nursing Sister (of QIDN)
QO₂ oxygen quotient
qod every other day
QP quanti-Pirquet (reaction)
qp *quantum placeat* (L) as much as you please
qpm every night
qq *quaque, quoque* (L) each, every, also
qqh *quaque quarta hora* (L) every four hours
qq hor *quaque hora* (L) every hour
QR *quantum rectum* (L) quantity is correct; quinaldine red
QRS Segment of electrocardiograph
QRZ *Quaddel Reaktion Zeit* (Ger) weal reaction time
QS quiet sleep
QS2 total electromechanical systole
qs *quantum satis* (L) sufficient quantity; *quantum sufficit* (L) as much as will suffice
q suff *quantum sufficit* (L) as much as will suffice
QT Quick's test (for pregnancy or for prothrombin)
qt quart
quadrupl *quadruplicato* (L) four times as much
qual quality, qualitative
qual anal qualitative analysis
quant quantity, quantitative
quant anal quantitative analysis
quar quarterly
quat *quattuor* (L) four
QUI Queen's University of Ireland
quing *quinque* (L) five
quint *quintus* (L) fifth
quor *quorum* (L) of which
quot *quoties* (L) as often as necessary
quotid *quotidie* (L) daily
qv *quantum vis* (L) as much as you wish; *quod vide* (L) which see

R

R any alkyl group of an alkane; Behnken's unit (of

roentgen-ray exposure); organic radical (in chemical formulas); race; racemic; radioactive mineral; radiology(-ologist); Rankine (temperature scale); reaction; reading; Réaumur (temperature scale); rectal; red; registered trademark; regulator (gene); *Reiz* (Ger) stimulus; relapse; relaxed; *remotum* (L) far; repressor; resazurin; resistance; resistant (with reference to disease); respiration; response; rest (in cell cycle); restricted; reverse Giemsa method; review; ribose; *Rickettsia;* right; right eye; roentgen; roentgenology (-ologist); rough (with reference to bacterial colonies); In formulas of amino acids, denotes characteristic side chain; Symbol for a gas constant (8.315 joules)

R factor   resistance factor (bacteriology)

+R   Rinne's test positive (test for hearing) (symbol for)

−R   Rinne's test negative (test for hearing) (symbol for)

RA   radioactive; ragweed antigen; Raynaud's phenomenon; repeat action; residual air; rheumatoid arthritis; right angle (angulation) (orthopaedics); right arm; right atrium; right auricle; robustrus archistriatalis (nucleus of brain)

Ra   radium

RAAMC   Royal Australian Army Medical Corps

RAC   Recombinant RNA Advisory Committee

rac   racemic

RAD   right axis deviation; roentgen administered dose

Rad   radiotherapy(-apist); radium

rad   radiation absorbed dose; radical; radius; *radix* (L) root

RADA   radioactive; right acromio-dorso-anterior (position of fetus); rosin amine-D-acetate

RADC   Royal Army Dental Corps

RADIO   radiotherapy

Radiol   Radiology(-ologist)

RADLCEN   Radiological Centre

RadLV   radiation leukaemia virus

RADP   right acromio-dorso-posterior (position of fetus)

RADWASTE   radioactive waste

RAFMS   Royal Air Force Medical Services

Ragg   rheumatoid agglutinator

RAHC   Royal Alexandra Hospital for Children (Camperdown NSW)

RAIU   radioactive iodine uptake

RAM   random access memory; Research Aviation Medicine

RAMC   Royal Army Medical Corps
RAP   renal artery pressure; right atrial pressure
rar   right arm reclining or recumbent
RAS   reticular activating system; rheumatoid arthritis serum (factor)
ras   *rasurae* (L) scrapings or filings
RAST   radio-allergosorbent test
RAT   repeat action tablet
RATG   rabbit antithymocyte globulin
RAV   Roux associated virus
RAVC   Royal Army Veterinary Corps
Raw   resistance, airway
RAZ   razoxane
Rb   rubidium
RBA   rescue breathing apparatus
RBBB   right bundle branch block
RBBsB   right bundle-branch system block
RBC   red blood cell count; red blood corpuscle (cell)
RBD   right border of dullness (of heart to percussion)
RBE   relative biological effectiveness (of radiation)
RBF   renal blood flow
Rb Imp   rubber base impression (dentistry)
RBN   retrobulbar neuritis
RBNA   Royal British Nurses Association
RBP   retinol-binding protein; riboflavine-binding protein
RBTC   Rational Behaviour Therapy Centre
RBZ   rubidazone (zorubicin)
RC   reaction centre; receptor-chemoeffector; red cell (corpuscle); Red Cross; referred care; respiration ceases; Respiratory Care; respiratory centre; rest cure; retention catheter; Roman Catholic; root canal
Rc   response, conditioned
RCA   red cell agglutination
RCAF   Royal Canadian Air Force
RCAMC   Royal Canadian Army Medical Corps
rCBF   regional cerebral blood flow
RCC   Radio-Chemical Centre; Radiological Control Centre; Rape Crisis Centre; receptor chemoeffector complex; renal cell carcinoma
RCCM   Regional Committee for Community Medicine (Brit)
RCD   relative cardiac dullness
RCDHS   Rehabilitation and Chronic Disease Hospital Section
RCF   relative centrifugal force

RCFR Red Cross Field Representative
RCGP Royal College of General Practitioners
RCHMS Regional Committee for Hospital Medical Services
RCI respiratory control index
RCM red cell mass; reinforced clostridial medium; replacement culture medium; right costal margin; Roux conditioned medium; Royal College of Midwives
RCN Royal College of Nursing
RCO aliphatic acyl radical
RCOG Royal College of Obstetricians and Gynaecologists
RCP riboflavine carrier protein; Royal College of Physicians
RCPath Royal College of Pathologists
RCPsych Royal College of Psychiatrists
RCPSGlas Royal College of Physicians and Surgeons, Glasgow
RCS reticulum cell sarcoma; Royal College of Science; Royal College of Surgeons
RCSE Royal College of Surgeons, Edinburgh
RCSI Royal College of Surgeons, Ireland
RCT randomized clinical trial; Rorschach Content Test
RCU Respiratory Care Unit
RCVS Royal College of Veterinary Surgeons
RD reaction of degeneration; registered dietitian; renal disease; retinal detachment; Reye's disease; rubber dam; ruptured disc
Rd reading
rd rutherford (unit of radioactivity)
R&D research and development
RDA recommended daily allowance; right dorsoanterior (position of fetus)
RdA reading age
RDC Research Diagnostic Criteria
RDE receptor destroying enzyme
RDH Registered Dental Hygienist
rDNA recombinant deoxyribonucleic acid
RDP right dorsoposterior (position of fetus)
RdQ reading quotient
RDS respiratory distress syndrome
RDT regular dialysis treatment; retinal damage threshold
RDW red cell size distribution width
RE radium emanation; rectal examination; resting energy; reticuloendothelium; retinol equivalent; right eye

REA Radiation Emergency Area; renal anastomosis
REACH Reassurance to Each (to help families of the mentally ill)
readm readmission
REAT Radiological Emergency Assistance Team
REB roentgen-equivalent biological
R-EBD-HS recessive-epidermolysis bullosa dystrophica-Hallopeau Siemens
rec *recens* (L) fresh; record; recreation; recurrent
RECG radioelectrocardiography
Recip recipient
Recomm recommendation
recond recondition(ing)
reconstr reconstruction
recryst recrystallize
rect *rectificatus* (L) rectified; rectum; rectus (muscle)
recur recurrent(-ence)
redig in pulv *redigatur in pulverem* (L) let it be reduced to powder
red in pulv *reductus in pulverem* (L) reduced to a powder
REDNP Regent's External Degree Nursing Program (New York)
redox reduction oxidation
REE rapid extinction effect
REEG radioelectroencephalograph
REF renal erythropoietic factor
ref refer(ence)
ref doc referring doctor
refl reflex
REFMS Recreation and Education for Multiple Sclerosis Victims
ref phys referring physician
REG Radiation Exposure Guide; radioencephalogram (-ograph)
Reg registered
reg regarding; region; regular
regen regenerate(-ation)
reg umb umbilical region
rehabil rehabilitation
REL rate of energy loss
rel related; relative
reliq *reliquus* (L) remainder
REM rapid eye movement (in sleep); roentgen equivalent man
rem roentgen equivalent man

REMAB   radiation equivalent manikin absorption
REMCAL   radiation equivalent manikin calibration
ren   *renovetur* (L) renew
ren sem   *renovetum seml* (L) shall be renewed only once
RET   right esotropia
ret   retired
retard   retarded (delayed)
retic count   reticulocyte count
retics   reticulocytes
rev   reverse; review; revolution
Rev of Sym   review of symptoms
RF   radial fibres (of the cochlea); receptive field (of visual cortex); Reitland-Franklin (unit); relative flow rate; releasing factor; replicative form; resistance factor; respiratory failure; reticular formation; rheumatic fever; rheumatoid factor; riboflavine
rf   radio frequency
R_F rate of flow (chromatography)
RFA   right frontoanterior (position of fetus)
RFC   rosette-forming cells
RFL   right frontolateral (position of fetus)
RFLS   rheumatoid-factor-like substance
RFN   Registered Fever Nurse
RFP   right frontoposterior (position of fetus)
RFPS (Glasgow)   Royal Faculty of Physicians and Surgeons of Glasgow
RFR   refraction
RFT   right frontotransverse (position of fetus)
R-G   Radiologist, General
Rg   Rodgers antibodies
RGC   retinal ganglial cells
RGE   relative gas expansion
RGN   Registered General Nurse
RGR   relative growth rate
RH   radiant heat; radiological health; relative humidity; releasing hormone; right hand; right hyperphoria; Royal Hospital (London); rheumatism
Rh   Rhesus (with reference to blood factors); *Rhipicephalus*
Rh−   Rhesus negative
Rh+   Rhesus positive
rh   *rhonchi* (L) râles
r/h   roentgens per hour
RHA   Regional Health Authority
RHA(T)   Regional Health Authority (Teaching) (Brit)

RHB Regional Hospital Board

RHC resin haemoperfusion column; respirations have ceased; right hypochondrium

RHCC/PP Reproductive Health Care Center/Planned Parenthood

RHCSA Regional Hospitals Consultants' and Specialists' Association

RHD Radiological Health Data; relative hepatic dullness; rheumatic heart disease

rheu fev rheumatic fever

rheu ht dis rheumatic heart disease

rheum rheumatic(-atism)

RHF right heart failure

RhIg rhesus immune globulin

Rhin rhinology(-ologist)

Rhiz *Rhizobium*

RHJSC Regional Hospital Junior Staff Committee (Brit)

RHM roentgen per hour at one metre

RhMK rhesus monkey kidney cells

r/hr roentgens per hour

RHS right hand side

RHU Registered Health Underwriter

RI radiation intensity; Recovery, Incorporated; refractive index; release-inhibiting; remission induction; replicative intermediate; respiratory illness; retroactive inhibition (psychology); retroactive interference; ribosome

RIA radio-immunoassay

RIA-DA radio-immunoassay double antibody (test)

RIC Royal Institute of Chemistry

RICM right intercostal margin

RID reversible intravas device

RIF release inhibiting factor; rifampicin; right iliac fossa

RIFC rat intrinsic factor concentrate

RIGH rabies immune globulin, human

RIH right inguinal hernia

RIHSA radioactive iodinated human serum albumin

RILT rabbit ileal loop test

RIM radioisotope medicine

RIMR Rockefeller Institute for Medical Research

RIPH Royal Institute of Public Health

RIPHH Royal Institute of Public Health and Hygiene

RIRB radioiodinated rose bengal

RISA radioactive iodinated serum albumin; radioimmunosorbent assay

RIT radio-iodinated triolein
RIV ramus interventricular
RKG radiocardiogram
RKY roentgen kymography
RL coarse râles (with reference to auscultation of chest); Radiation Laboratory; reduction level (the reciprocal of respiratory quotient); reticular lamina; right lower; Ringer lactate; Royal Licence (Brit); stimulus (*Reiz*) limen
RL$_3$ many coarse râles
Rl medium râles
Rl$_2$ moderate number of medium râles
rl fine râles
rl$_1$ few fine râles
RLBCD right lower border of cardiac dullness
RLC residual lung capacity
RLD related living donor; ruptured lumbar disc
RLE right lower extremity
RLF retrolental fibroplasia; right lateral femoral (site of injection)
RLL right lower lobe (of lung)
RLMD rat liver mitochondria (and submitochondrial particles derived by) digitonin (treatment)
RLND regional lymph node dissection
RLQ right lower quadrant (of abdomen)
RLR right lateral rectus (muscle of eye)
RLS A person who stammers having difficulty in enunciating R, L, and S
RM radical mastectomy; range of movement (motion); red marrow; respiratory movement
Rm remission
RMA Registered Medical Assistant; relative medullary area (of the kidney); right mentoanterior (position of fetus)
RMAC Regional Medical Advisory Committee (Brit)
RMBF regional myocardial blood flow
RMD retromanubrial dullness
RMK rhesus monkey kidney
RML right mediolateral (episiotomy); right middle lobe (of lungs)
RMM rapid micromedia method
RMN Registered Mental Nurse (England and Wales)
RMO Regional Medical Officer; Resident Medical Officer
RMP Regional Medical Program; rifampicin; right

mentoposterior (position of fetus)

RMPA Royal Medico-Psychological Association

RMR right medial rectus (muscle of eye)

RMS respiratory muscle strength

RMSF Rocky Mountain spotted fever

RMT relative medullary thickness (of kidney); right mentotransverse (position of fetus)

RMV respiratory minute volume

RN radionuclide; red nucleus; Registered Nurse; Royal Navy

Rn radon

RNA Registered Nurse Anesthetist; ribonucleic acid; rough, non-capsulated avirulent (with reference to bacteria)

RND radical neck dissection

RNIB Royal National Institute for the Blind

RNID Royal National Institute for the Deaf

RNm red nucleus, magnocellular division

RNMD Registered Nurse for Mental Defectives

RNMS Registered Nurse for Mentally Subnormal

RNP ribonucleoprotein

Rnt roentgenology(-ologist)

RO reverse osmosis; routine order

R/O rule out

ROA right occipitoanterior (position of fetus)

ROC residual organic carbon

Roent roentgenology(-ologist)

ROL right occipitolateral (position of fetus)

ROM range of movement (motion); read only memory; rupture of membranes

ROP right occipitoposterior (position of fetus)

Ror Rorschach (test)

ROS review of systems

ROT remedial occupational therapy; right occipitotransverse (position of fetus)

rot rotation, rotator

rout routine

RP radial pulse; refractory period; respiratory rate, pulse rate (index); retinitis pigmentosa; retrograde pyelography; retroperitoneal; ribose phosphate; ristocetin polymyxin

R-P Radiologist – paediatric

RPA resultant physiological acceleration; reverse passive anaphylaxis

RPC reticularis pontis caudalis

RPCF Reiter protein complement fixation (test)
RPE retinal pigment epithelium
RPF relaxed pelvic floor; renal plasma flow
RPG radiation protection guide
RPGMEC Regional Postgraduate Medical Educational Committee
RPGG retroplacental gamma globulin
RPGN rapidly progressive glomerular nephritis
RPh Registered Pharmacist
RPHA reverse passive haemagglutination
RP-HPLC reversed phase – high performance liquid chromatography
RPI reticulocyte production index
RPLAD retroperitoneal lymphoadenectomy
RPLC reversed-phase liquid chromatography
rpm revolutions per minute
RPMI Roswell Park Memorial Institute
RPP retropubic prostatectomy
RPPI role perception picture inventory
RPPR red cell precursor production rate
RPR rapid plasma reagin (test)
RPS renal pressor substance
rps revolutions per second
RPT Registered Physical Therapist
Rpt repeat; report
RPTD ruptured
RQ recovery quotient; respiratory quotient
R&R rate and rhythm (of pulse)
RR radiation reaction (cells); radiation response; recovery response; relative response; relative risk; respiratory rate; risk ratio; Riva-Rocci (sphygmomanometer)
RRA radioreceptor assay
RRC routine respiratory care; Royal Red Cross
RR&E round, regular and equal (with reference to pupils of eyes)
RRL Registered Record Librarian
rRNA ribosomal ribonucleic acid
RRP relative refractory period
RRT Registered Respiratory Therapist; resazurin reduction time
RS *Rauwolfia serpentina;* reading of standard; recipient's serum; rectal sinus; reducing sugar; reinforcing stimulus; renal specialist; resorcinol-sulphur; respiratory syncytial (virus); response to stimulus (ratio); review of symptoms; Reye's syndrome; right sacrum; right side;

Ringer's solution

RSA rabbit serum albumin; relative standard accuracy; right sacroanterior (position of fetus)

RSB Regimental Stretcher-Bearer; reticulocyte standard buffer

RSC reversible sickled cell; right-side colon cancer

RScA right scapuloanterior

rsch research

RSCN Registered Sick Children's Nurse

RScP right scapuloposterior (position of fetus)

RSD reflex sympathetic dystrophy

RSE reverse sutured eye

RSES Rosenberg Self-Esteem Scale

RSH Royal Society of Health

RSIC Radiation Shielding Information Center

RSIVP rapid sequence intravenous pyelogram

RSL right sacrolateral (position of fetus)

RSM Royal Society of Medicine

RSNA Radiological Society of North America

RSO Resident Surgical Officer

RSP right sacroposterior (position of fetus)

RSPCA Royal Society for the Prevention of Cruelty to Animals

RSPH Royal Society for the Promotion of Health

RSPK recurrent spontaneous psychokinesis

RSR regular sinus rhythm

RSSE Russian spring-summer encephalitis

RST radiosensitivity testing; right sacrotransverse (position of fetus)

RSTMH Royal Society of Tropical Medicine and Hygiene

RSV respiratory syncytial virus; Rous sarcoma virus

RT radiologic technologist; radiotherapy; radium therapy; rational therapy; reaction time; reading test; recreational therapy; reduction time; Registered Technician (American Registry of X-ray Technicians); resistance transfer; respiratory therapy; room temperature

Rt rotundus nucleus

rt right

RTA renal tubule acidosis; road traffic accident

Rtd retarded; retired

RTF resistance transfer factor; respiratory tract fluid

RTI respiratory tract infection

rtl rectal

R test reductase test

RTR Recreational Therapist Registered; red blood cell turnover rate

RU rat unit; reading of unknown; resin uptake; right upper; Roentgen unit

rub *ruber* (L) red

RUE right upper extremity

RUI Royal University of Ireland

RUL right upper eyelid; right upper lobe (of lung)

RUO right ureteral orifice

RUOQ right upper outer quadrant (site of injection)

rupt rupture(d)

RUQ right upper quadrant

RV reinforcement value; residual volume; retroversion; right ventricle; rubella vaccine

RVA renal vascular resistance

RVD relative vertebral density

RVEDV right ventricle end-diastolic volume

RVESV right ventricular end-systolic volume

RVG right visceral ganglion

RVH renovascular hypertension; right ventricular hypertrophy

RVLG right ventrolateral gluteal (site of injection)

RVO Regional Veterinary Officer; relaxed vaginal outlet

RV/RA renal vein/renal activity (ratio)

RVS relative value scale or schedule; reported visual sensation

RVSW right ventricular stroke work

RW radiological warfare

R-W Rideal-Walker (phenol coefficient test)

Rx prescription; *recipe* (L) take; treatment or therapy

RXLI recessive X-linked ichthyosis

RXT right exotropia

RxTV Prescription Television

S

S sacral (in vertebral formulas); saline; saturated, saturation; same; section; sedimentation coefficient; senile; sensation; sensitive; *signa, signetur* (L) write, let it be written, label; silicate; single (marital status); singular; small; smooth (with reference to colonies of bacteria); soft (with reference to diet); solid; soluble; solute;

space; special preparations necessary for test; spherical; spherical lens; stimulus; subject (of an experiment); substrate; sulphur; supravergence; surface; surgeon, surgery; Svedberg (unit of sedimentation coefficient); synthesis (of DNA in cell cycle)

s scruple (apothecaries); second (unit of time) (SI); section; see; *semis* (L) half; sensation; series; sign(ed); singular; *sinister* (L) left; son

Σ sigma; sum; euphemistic abbreviation for syphilis

s- symmetric isomer

s *sine* (L) without

S1, S2, etc first sacral nerve, second sacral nerve, etc

S$_1$, S$_2$, S$_3$, S$_4$ first, second, third and fourth heart sounds

S$_x$ symptoms or signs

SA salicylic acid; salt added; sarcoma; Schizophrenics Anonymous; *secundum artem* (L) according to the art; self-analysis; semen analysis; serum albumin; sex appeal; soluble in alkaline solution; specific activity; standard accuracy; *Staphylococcus aureus;* surface antigen; surface area; sustained action (with reference to drugs)

S-A sino-atrial (node); sino-auricular

sa *secundum artem* (L) according to art, by skill

S&A Sickness and Accident (Insurance); sugar and acetone

SAA serum amyloid-A (protein)

SAB Sabouraud (dextrose agar); Society of American Bacteriologists

SABHI Sabouraud dextrose agar and brain heart infusion

SABP spontaneous acute bacterial peritonitis

SAC saccharine

sacc cogwheel (respiration)

SACE serum angiotensin converting enzyme (activity)

SACH Small Animal Care Hospital

SAD sugar, acetone, diacetic acid (test)

SADS Schedule for Affective Disorders and Schizophrenia

SAFA soluble antigen fluorescent antibody (test)

SAG salicyl acyl glucuronide

SAH subarachnoid haemorrhage

SAI Self-Analysis Inventory

SAICAR succinoamino-imidazole-carboxide

Sal *Salmonella*

sal salicylate; *secundum artis legis* (L) according to the rules of art

salicyl salicylate
Salm *Salmonella*
SAM scanning acoustic microscope; sex arousal mechanism
SAMA Student American Medical Association
SAMI socially acceptable monitoring instrument
SAN sinoatrial node
Sanat sanatorium
sanit sanitarium; sanitation(-itary)
SAP serum amyloid-P; *Staphylococcus aureus* protease
sapon saponification
SAR sexual attitude reassessment; structure activity relationship (dentistry)
Sar sulpharsphenamine
SAS sterile aqueous suspension
SAT satellite; School Ability Test (psychology); *sine acido thymonucleinico* (L) without thymonucleic acid
sat saturated
sat'd saturated
SATL surgical Achilles tendon lengthening
satn saturation
sat sol saturated solution
SAU statistical analysis unit
SB Bachelor of Science; shortness of breath; sick bay; sinus bradycardia; Stanford-Binet (intelligence test); stillbirth; stretcher-bearer
Sb *stibium* (L) antimony; strabismus
SBA sick bay attendant (Navy); soy bean agglutinin
SBE breast self-examination; shortness of breath on exertion; subacute bacterial endocarditis
SBF serologic-blocking factor
SBG selenite brilliant green
SBH sea blue histiocytosis
SBN$_2$ single-breath nitrogen (test)
SBNS Society of British Neurological Surgeons
SBOM soy bean oil meal
SBP steroid-binding plasma (protein); systolic blood pressure
SBR strict bed rest; styrene-butadiene rubber
SBStJ Serving Brother, Order of St John of Jerusalem
SBT serum bacteriological titres
SBTI soy bean trypsin inhibitor
SC closure of semilunar valves; sacrococcygeal; Sanitary Corps; Schwann cell; sciatic nerve; science, scientific; *scilicet* (L) namely; *scrupulus* (L) scruple; secretory

component; self-care; service connected; sex chromatin; sick call; sickle cell; silicone coated; skin conductance; slow component (neurology); squamous cancer; Stepped Care; stimulus, conditioned; subcutaneous; sugar coated

S-C sickle cell haemoglobin C disease

Sc scapula

sc without correction

SCA sickle cell anaemia; sperm-coating antigen

SCAA Skin Care Association of America

SCAN scantiscan; suspected child abuse and neglect

Scand Scandinavian

SCAT School and College Ability test; sheep-cell agglutination test

scat *scatula* (L) box

scat orig *scatula originalis* (L) original package: manufacturer's package and label

SCB strictly confined to bed

SCC Services for Crippled Children; short course chemotherapy; squamous cell carcinoma

SCCL small cell (oat cell) carcinoma of the lung

SCCM Sertoli cell culture medium

SCD sickle cell disease; subacute combined degeneration (of spinal cord); sudden cardiac death

ScD Doctor of Science

ScDA *scapuladextra anterior* (L) right scapuloanterior (position of fetus)

ScDP *scapuladextra posterior* (L) right scapuloposterior (position of fetus)

SCE secretory carcinoma of the endometrium; sister chromatid exchange

SCF Skin Cancer Foundation

SCG sodium cromoglycate

SChE serum cholinesterase

SCI Science Citation Index; Science of Creative Intelligence (Transcendental Meditation); spinal cord injury

Sci science; scientific

SCID severe combined immune deficiency

SCIPP sacrococcygeal to inferior pubic point

SCIS spinal cord injury service

SCL scleroderma

ScLA *scapulolaeva anterior* (L) left scapuloanterior (position of fetus)

Scler sclerosis

ScLP *scapulolaeva posterior* (L) left scapuloposterior

(position of fetus)

SCM State Certified Midwife; streptococcal cell membrane

SCMO Senior Clerical Medical Officer

SCN potassium thiocyanate

SCND thiocyanate

SCNS subcutaneous nerve stimulation

SCOP scopolamine (hyoscine)

scp spherical candle power

SCR skin conductance response

SCr serum creatinine

scr scruple

SCRAP Simple Complex Reaction-Time Apparatus

SCS Society of Clinical Surgery

SCT sugar-coated tablet

SCU Special Care Unit

SCUBA self-contained underwater breathing apparatus

SCV smooth, capsulated, virulent (with reference to bacteria)

SD septal defect; serologically determined; serologically defined; skin destruction; skin dose; spontaneous delivery; standard deviation; stone disintegration; streptodornase; sudden death; systolic discharge

S-D sickle cell haemoglobin D (disease)

Sd stimulus drive (psychology)

S^d stimulus, discriminative

SDA *sacrodextra anterior* (L) right sacroanterior (position of fetus); specific dynamic action (of foods); succinic dehydrogenase activity

SDAT senile dementia Alzheimer type

SDC sodium deoxycholate; succinyldicholine

SDE specific dynamic effect

SDF slow death factor

SDH sorbitol dehydrogenase; spinal dorsal horn

SDHD sudden death heart disease

SDI standard deviation interval

SDM sensory detection method

SDN sexually dimorphic nucleus

SDP *sacrodextra posterior* (L) right sacroposterior (position of fetus)

SDS School Dental Service; sexual differentiation scale; sodium dodecyl sulphate; Specific Diagnosis Service; sudden death syndrome

Sds sounds

SDT *sacrodextra transversa* (L) right sacrotransverse

(position of fetus)

SE saline enema; sanitary engineering; solid extract; sphenoethmoidal (suture); spherical equivalent; stage of exhaustion (in GAS); standard error

Se selenium

SEA sheep erythrocyte agglutination (test); spontaneous electrical activity (physiology); staphylococcal enterotoxin A

SEB staphylococcal enterotoxin B

SEBA staphylococcal enterotoxin B antiserum

SEBM Society of Experimental Biology and Medicine

SEC *secundum* (L) according to; soft elastic capsules

sec second (unit of time); secondary; secretary; section(s)

sect section

SED skin erythema dose; spondyloepiphyseal dysplasia; staphylococcal enterotoxin D

sed *sedes* (L) stool; sedimentation

SEER surveillance, epidemiology and end-result reporting

SEF somatically evoked field

SEG sonoencephalogram

segm segmented

segs segmented neutrophils (polymorphonuclear leucocytes)

SEH Société Européenne d'Hématologie

SEM scanning electron microscope; secondary enrichment medium; standard error of mean

sem *semen* (L) seed; *semi, semis* (L) one-half; seminal

semidr *semidrachma* (L) half a drachm

semih *semihora* (L) half an hour

sem vcs seminal vesicle

SEN State Enrolled Nurse

sen sensitive

SENS sensitivities test

SEP *sepultus* (L) buried; somatosensory evoked potential; sperm entry point; systolic ejection period

separ *separatum* (L) separately

sept *septem* (L) seven

seq *sequela* (L) that which follows

seq luce *sequenti luce* (L) the following day

SER service; somatosensory evoked response

sER smooth endoplasmic reticulum

Ser serine

ser series, serial

ser sect serial sections

serv *serva* (L) keep, preserve; services

SERVHEL Service and Health Record

SES Society of Eye Surgeons; socioeconomic status; spatial emotional stimuli

sesquih *sesquihora* (L) an hour and a half

sex sexual

s expr *sine expressione* (L) without expressing or pressing

SF safety factor; scarlet fever; seminal fluid; serum fibrinogen; sodium azide, faecal (medium); spinal fluid; sterile female; *Streptococcus faecalis;* stress formula; sulphation factor (of blood serum); Sweberg flotation (unit); synovial fluid

SFC soluble fibrin-fibrinogen complex; spinal fluid count

SFFF sedimentation field flow fractionization

SFGS stratum fibrosum et griseum superficiale

SFL Sexual Freedom League

SFO subfornical organ

SFP stopped flow pressure

SFW shell fragment wound

SG Sachs-Georgi (test); soluble gelatin (with reference to capsules); Surgeon General

sg specific gravity

SGA small for gestational age

SGC spermicide-germicide compound

SGM Society for General Microbiology

SGO Surgeon General's Office

SGOT serum glutamic oxalo-acetic transaminase

SGP Society of General Physiologists

SGPT serum glutamic pyruvic transaminase

SGR submandibular gland renin

S-Gt Sachs-Georgi test

SGV salivary gland virus

SH serum hepatitis; sexual harassment; sick in hospital; social history; somatotrophic (growth) hormone; spontaneously hypertensive; sulphydryl; surgical history

Sh sheep (in veterinary medicine); *Shigella* (bacteriology)

sh short; shoulder

S&H speech and hearing

SHAA serum hepatitis associated antigen; Society of Hearing Aid Audiologists

SHAA-Ab serum hepatitis associated antigen-antibody

SHA-Ab serum hepatitis associated antibody

SHARP School Health Additional Referral Program

SHB subacute hepatitis with bridging

Try tryptophan
TS temperature sensitive; temporal stem; Teratology Society; terminal (or greater) sensation; test solution; thoracic surgery; total solids; Tourette syndrome; toxic substance; transsexual; transverse section; transverse tubular system; tricuspid stenosis; triple strength; tuberous sclerosis; tubular (tracheal) sound; tumour specific; type-specific antibodies
T/S thyroid: serum (radioiodide ratio)
TSA tumour specific antigen; toluene sulphonic acid (test)
TSC tryptose-sulphite cyclosterone (agar)
TSD target skin distance
TSE testicular self-examination
T sect transverse or cross section
T-set tracheotomy set
TSF thrombopoietic stimulating factor; triceps skinfold
TSH thyroid-stimulating (thyrotrophic) hormone
TSH-RF thyroid-stimulating hormone-releasing factor
TSI thyroid-stimulating immunoglobulin; triple sugar (lactose, glucose, sucrose), iron (agar)
TSIA triple sugar iron agar
TSM type-specific M (protein)
TSN tryptophan peptone sulphide neomycin (agar)
TSP total serum protein
tsp teaspoon
TSR testosterone sterilized (female) rat
TSS toxic shock syndrome
TSSU theatre sterile supply unit
TST treadmill stress testing
TSTA tumour specific transplantation antigen
TSU triple sugar urea (agar)
TT tablet triturate; tetanus toxoid; tetrathionate (broth); thrombin time; thymol turbidity; tibial tubercle; total thyroxine; transit time (of blood through heart and lungs); tuberculin tested (milk)
T&T time and temperature
TTA transtracheal aspiration
TTC triphenyltetrazolium chloride
TTGA tellurite-taurocholate-gelatin agar
TTH thyrotrophic hormone (*see* TSH)
TTO to take out
TTP thrombotic thrombocytopenic purpura; thymidine triphosphate
TTPA triethylene thiophosphoramide (thiotepa)

SP sacrum to pubis; Schwangerschaftsprotein; standard practice; standard procedure; staphylococcal protein A; stool preservative (Hajna); subliminal perception; substance P (a peptide); suprapubic

S/P status post

Sp spine (esp. spine of scapula); *Spirillum;* summation potential

sp space; species; specific; spinal; *spiritus* (L) spirit

SPA suprapubic aspiration

SPAM scanning photo-acoustic microscopy

Span Spanish

SPC salicylamide, phenacetin, and caffeine; standard plate count

SPCA serum prothrombin conversion accelerator (Factor VII) (proconvertin)

sp cd spinal cord

spec special; specialist; specific; specimen

specif specification

SPF skin protection factor; specific pathogen free; spectrophotofluorometer

sp fl spinal fluid

sp gr specific gravity

SPH severely and profoundly handicapped

Sph sphingomyelin

sph spherical; spherical lens

sp ht specific heat

SPI serum precipitable iodine

sp indet *species indeterminata* (L) species indeterminate

sp inquir *species inquirendae* (L) species of doubtful status

spir spiral; spiritual; *spiritus* (L) spirit

spiss *spissus* (L) dried

SPK Spinnbarkeit (with reference to cervical mucus)

SPL skin potential level; sound pressure level

SPM suspended particulate matter

SpM spiriformis medialis (nucleus)

SPMB strong partial maternal behaviour

SPN sympathetic preganglionic neuron

sp n *species novum* (L) new species

sp nov *species novum* (L) new species

spon spontaneous

SPP Sexuality Preference Profile; suprapubic prostatectomy

spp species (plural)

SPPS stable plasma protein solution

SPR serial probe recognition; Society for Pediatric Radiology; Society for Pediatric Research; Society for Psychical Research

SPRIA solid phase radioimmunoassay

SPRU Science Policy Research Unit (Univ of Sussex)

SPS Society of Pelvic Surgeons; sulphite polymyxin; sulphadiazine (agar)

spt *spiritus* (L) spirit

SPU Society of Pediatric Urology

SPV Shope papilloma virus

SQ subcutaneous; Sick Quarters (Brit)

sq square

sq cell ca squamous cell carcinoma

sqq *sequentia* (L) and following

SQUID superconducting quantum interference device

SQ3R survey, question, read, review, recite (psychology)

SR sarcoplasmic reticulum; secretion rate; sedimentation rate; seizure resistant; senior; Senior Registrar; sensitization response; sex ratio; sigma reaction; sinus rhythm; soluble, repository (with reference to penicillin); spontaneous discharge rate; stage of resistance (in general adaptation syndrome); stimulus-response; stomach rumble; sulphonamide resistant; systems review

Sr strontium

^{85}Sr radioactive strontium

SRaw specific resistance, airway

SRBC sheep red blood cells

SR cells sensitization response cells (in vaginal smears)

SRD Society for the Relief of Distress; Society for the Right to Die; soluble, repository, plus dihydrostreptomycin (with reference to penicillin)

SRF skin respiratory factor; somatotrophin-releasing factor

SRH single radial haemolysis; spontaneously responding hyperthyroidism

SRHL Southwestern Radiological Health Laboratory

SRI severe renal insufficiency

SRN State Registered Nurse

sRNA soluble ribonucleic acid

SRNS steroid-responsive nephrotic syndrome

SRP State Registered Physiotherapist; Society for Radiological Protection

SRS Silver-Russell syndrome; slow reacting substance; Social and Rehabilitation Service (HHS)

SRS-A slow reacting substance of anaphylaxis

SRT Science, Research, Technology; sedimentation rate test; simple reaction time; sinus node recovery time; social relations test; speech reception threshold

SR-RSV Schmidt-Ruppin strain Rous sarcoma virus

SS saline soak; saliva sample; saturated solution; serum sickness; seizure sensitive; *Shigella* and *Salmonella* (agar); single-stranded (DNA); Sjögren's syndrome; soap suds; sparingly soluble; standard score (psychology); sterile solution; suction socket

ss *sensu stricto* (L) in the strict sense

ss (s̄s̄) *semis* (L) one half

SSA skin-sensitizing antibodies; Social Security Administration; Smith surface antigen

SSCQT Selective Service College Qualifying Test

SSCr stainless steel crown (dentistry)

SSD source-skin distance

SSE skin self-examination; soapsuds enema

SSI supplemental security income; System Sign Inventory

SSIDS siblings of sudden infant death syndrome (victims)

SSM sesquiterpenoid stress metabolites; subsynaptic membrane

SSO Society of Surgical Oncology

SSP supersensitivity perception

SSPE subacute sclerosing panencephalitis

SSPL saturation sound pressure level

SSS sick sinus syndrome; specific soluble substance (polysaccharide hapten); sterile saline soak

sss *stratum super stratum* (L) layer upon layer

SSStJ Serving Sister, Order of St John of Jerusalem

s str *sensu stricto* (L) in the strict sense

SSU self-service unit

ssv *sub signo veneni* (L) under a poison label

SSX sulfisoxazole (sulphafurazole)

ST esotropia (with l or r); heat-stable (enterotoxin); sedimentation time; skin test; slight trace; standardized test (psychology); station; stimulus; stress testing; surface tension; survival time

S-T sickle-cell thalassaemia

ST 37 hexylresorcinol

St subtype

st *stet, stent* (L) let it stand, let them stand

stabs band cells (non-segmented polymorphonuclear leucocytes)

standard   standardization(-ized)
StanPsych   Standard Psychiatric (nomenclature)
Staph   *Staphylococcus*
stat   *statim* (L) at once, immediately; statistics
Stb   stillborn
STD   sexually transmitted disease; skin test dose; standard test dose
std   standard(-ized)
Stereo   stereogram
STH   somatotrophic (growth) hormone
STI   serum trypsin inhibitor
STIA   Scientific, Technological, and International Affairs
stillat   *stillatim* (L) by drops or in small quantities
stillb   stillborn
stimn   stimulation
STL   swelling, tenderness, limitation (of movement)
STM   scanning tunneling microscope; short-term memory
STN   subthalamic nucleus
STP   Hallucinogen of which DOM is the active principle; standard (normal) temperature and pulse; standard temperature and pressure
STPD   standard temperature and pressure, dry
Strep   *Streptococcus*
struct   structural
STS   serological test for syphilis; standard test for syphilis
STSA   Southern Thoracic Surgical Association
STT   sensitization test; standard triple therapy (for hypertension)
STU   skin test unit
STZ   streptozocin
SU   salicyluric acid; sensation unit; Sigma units; strontium unit; sulphonamide
su   *sumat* (L) let him take
SUA   serum uric acid
subac   subacute
subcrep   subcrepitant
subcut   subcutaneous(ly)
sub fin coct   *sub finem coctionis* (L) towards the end of boiling
subling   sublingual
submand   submandibular
subq   subcutaneous (injection)
subsp   subspecies
substd   substandard

suc   *succus* (L) juice
Succ   succinate
suf   sufficient
sulph   sulphate
sulpha   sulphonamide
sum   *sume, sumantur* (L) take, let it be taken
sum tal   *sumat talem* (L) take one like this
SUN   Standard Units and Nomenclature; serum urea nitrogen
sup   superior; supination; supine; *supra* (L) above, superior
supp   suppository
suppl   supplement(ary)
suppos   suppository
supra cit   *supra citato* (L) cited above
supt   superintendent
Surg   surgeon; surgery, surgical
SUS   supressor sensitive
susp   suspension
SUV   sociated unilamellar vesicles
SV   sarcoma virus; satellite virus; scalp vein; simian virus; sinus venosus; snake venom; stimulus value; stroke volume
S/V   surface to volume ratio
Sv   Sievert unit (100 rems)
sv   single vibrations; *spiritus vini* (L) alcoholic spirit
SVC   superior vena cava
SVCP   Special Virus Cancer Program
SVCS   superior vena cava syndrome
SVI   stroke volume index
SVR   systemic vascular resistance
svr   *spiritus vini rectificatus* (L) rectified spirit of wine, alcohol
SVT   supraventricular tachycardia
svt   *spiritus vini tenuis* (L) proof spirit
SW   seriously wounded; slow wave; Social Worker; sterile water
Sw   swine (in veterinary medicine)
SWA   seriously wounded in action
SWD   short wave diathermy
SWE   slow wave encephalography
SWI   sterile water for injection; stroke work index
SWIM   sperm washing insemination method
SWR   serum Wassermann reaction
SWS   slow wave sleep

Sx   symptoms or signs
SXT   sulphamethoxazole
SY   syphilis
sym   symmetry, symmetrical; symptoms
symb   symbol(ic)
sympath   sympathetic
sympt   symptoms
SYN   synthetic
syn   synonym
synd   syndrome
synth   synthetic
syph   syphilis; syphilology(-ologist)
syr   *syrupus* (L) syrup
sys   system(ic)
syst   systemic; systolic
syst m   systolic murmur
SZ   streptozocin
Sz   seizure; skin impedance

T

T   tamoxifen; tau; temperature; temporary; tension (esp. intraocular); tera (prefix) (SI); term; tetracycline; thoracic; thymine; thymus-derived (lymphocyte); thyroid; tidal gas (respiration); topical (with reference to administration of drugs); total; toxicity; transition point; transmittance (symbol for, in spectrophotometry); transverse; tumour; type
t   temporal; *ter* (L) three times; terminal; time; translocation
τ tau; Symbol for life(time) of radioactive isotope
$T_{1/2}$ Symbol for half-life(time) of radioactive isotope
T_1, T_2, **etc**   first thoracic vertebra, second thoracic vertebra, etc.
T_3 triiodothyronine
T_4 thyroxine
T+1, T+2, etc   Symbols indicating stages of increased intraocular tension
T−1, T−2, etc   Symbols indicating stages of decreased intraocular tension
T-1824   Evans blue
TA   Teaching Assistant; temperature, axillary; thermo-

philic *Actinomyces;* total alkaloids; toxin-antitoxin; Transactional Analysis; transaldolase; transplantation antigen; tricuspid atresia; true anomaly; tryptophane acid (reaction); tryptose agar; tuberculin, alkaline; tumour-associated

T&A tonsillectomy and adenoidectomy; tonsillitis and adenoiditis; tonsils and adenoids

TAAF thromboplastic activity of amniotic fluid

TAB typhoid, paratyphoid A, and paratyphoid B (vaccine)

tab *tabella* (L) a tablet

TABC total aerobic bacteria count; typhoid-paratyphoid A, B and C (vaccine)

TABT combined TAB vaccine, tetanus toxoid

TABTD combined TAB vaccine, tetanus toxoid and diphtheria toxoid

TAF toxoid-antitoxin floccules; *Tuberculin Albumosefrei* (Ger) albumose-free tuberculin; tumour angiogenesis factor

TAG thymine, adenine, guanine

TAH total abdominal hysterectomy; total artificial heart

tal *talis* (L) such a one

T-ALL T-cell acute lymphoblastic leukaemia

TAM tamoxifen; thermoacidurans agar modified; toxoid-antitoxin mixture

TAMIS Telemetric Automated Microbial Identification System

TAN total ammonia nitrogen

tan tangent

TANS Territorial Army Nursing Service

TAO triacetyloleandomycin

TAR thrombocytopenia with absent radii

T'ASE tryptophane synthetase

TAT tetanus antitoxin; Thematic Apperception Test; toxin-antitoxin

TB thromboxane B; thymol blue; total base; tracheal bronchiolar (region); tracheobronchitis; trapezoid body; tubercle bacillus; tuberculosis

TBA tertiary butyl acetate; thiobarbituric acid; to be added; tubercle bacillus; tuberculosis

TBB transbronchial biopsy

TBBM total body bone mineral

TBE tick-borne encephalitis; tuberculin bacillen emulsion

TBG testosterone-binding globulin; thyroxine-binding

globulin

TBGP total blood granulocyte pool

TBI tooth brushing instruction (dentistry); total body irradiation

TBLC term birth, living child

TBM tuberculous meningitis

TBP testosterone-binding protein; thyroxine-binding protein; tributyl phosphate

TBPA thyroxine-binding prealbumin

TBS total body solute

tbs tablespoon

TBSA total body surface area

tbsp tablespoon

TB-Vis isoniazid

TBW total body water; total body weight

TC tetracycline; thermal conductivity; thoracic cage; thyrocalcitonin; tissue culture; to contain; total cholesterol; total colonoscopy; transcobalamin; transcutaneous; tuberculin, contagious; type and crossmatch

Tc technetium

T&C turn and cough

TCA tricalcium aluminate; tricarboxylic acid (cycle); trichloroacetate; trichloroacetic acid; tricyclic antidepressant

TCAP trimethyl-cetyl-ammonium pentachlorphenate (a fungicide)

TCB tumour cell burden

TCBS thiosulphate citrate bile salt sucrose (agar)

TCC thromboplastic cell component

TCD tissue culture dose

TCE tetrachloro-diphenyl-ethane (a mosquito larvicide); trichloroethanol

TCES transcutaneous cranial electrical stimulation

TCESOM trichlorethylene-extracted soybean-oil meal

TCGF thymus cell growth factor (interleukin 2)

TCH turn, cough, hyperventilate

Tchg teaching

Tchr teacher

TCI to come in (to hospital)

TCID tissue culture infective dose

TCID$_{50}$ median tissue culture infective dose

T-CLL T-cell chronic lymphatic leukaemia

TCM tissue culture medium

TCP trichlorophenol; tricreslyl phosphate (an antiesterase)

TCR thalamocortical relay

TCT calcitonin; thyrocalcitonin

TCu copper T (an IUD)

TCV thoracic cage volume

TD temporary disability; tetanus and diphtheria (toxoids); thoracic duct; threshold dose; thymus dependent (cells); timed disintegration; to deliver; torsion dystonia; total disability; total dose (of radiation); treating distance; treatment or therapy discontinued; tuberoinfundibular dopaminergic; typhoid-dysentery

td *ter die* (L) three times daily

TDD Telecommunication Device for the Deaf; tetradecadiene; thoracic duct drainage; Tuberculous Diseases Diploma

TDE tetrachlorodiphenylethane (an insecticide); total digestible energy

TDI Therapy Dogs International

TDL thoracic duct lymph or lymphocytes; thymus dependent lymphocytes

TDN total digestible nutrients

T-DNA transferred deoxyribonucleic acid

TDS temperature, depth, salinity; temperature-determined sex

tds *ter die sumendum* (L) to be taken three times a day

TDT thermal death time; tone decay test

TDZ thymus-dependent zone (of lymph node)

TE Teacher of Electrotherapy; tetracycline; thromboembolism; tracheoesophageal; trial (and) error

Te tellurium; tetanus

T-e *see* ET-3

TEA tetraethylammonium

TEAB tetraethylammonium bromide

TEAC tetraethylammonium chloride

TEC transient erythroblastopenia of childhood

T&EC Trauma and Emergency Center

tech technical

TED threshold erythema dose

TEE tyrosine ethyl ester

TEM transmission electron microscope

temp temperature; temporal; temporary

temp dext *tempus dextro* (L) to the right temple

temp sinist *tempus sinistro* (L) to the left temple

TEN total excretory (or excreted) nitrogen; toxic epidermal necrolysis

TER total endoplasmic reticulum; transcapillary escape

route

ter *tere* (L) rub; tertiary

Terleu tertiary leucine

term terminal

ter sim *tere simul* (L) tub together

TES transcutaneous electrical stimulation; transmural electrical stimulation

TET Teacher of Electrotherapy

tet tetanus

TETRAC tetraiodothyroacetic acid

TEV talipes equinovarus

TF tactile fremitus; temperature factor; thymidine factor; transfer factor; transferrin; tuberculin filtrate; tuning fork

TFA total fatty acids

TFC transferrin, common form

TFN total faecal nitrogen

TFNS Territorial Force Nursing Service

TF/P tubular fluid plasma

TFR total fertility rate

TFS testicular feminization syndrome

TG tetraglycine; thioglycolate broth; thioguanine; thromboglobulin; thyroglobulin; triglyceride

Tg generation time; type genus

TGA taurocholate gelatin agar; total glycoalkaloids; transient global amnesia; transposition of great arteries

TGE transmissible gastroenteritis; tryptone glucose extract (broth or agar)

TGF transforming growth factor

TGG turkey gamma globulin

TGT thromboplastin generation test or time

TGY tryptone (tryptophane peptone) glucose yeast (agar)

TH tetrahydrocortisol; thyroid hormone (thyroxine)

Th thenar; thorax, thoracic; thorium

THA tetrahydroaminoacridine

ThA thoracic aorta

THC tetrahydrocannabinol; tetrahydrocortisol; thiocarbanidin

THE tetrahydrocortisone or tetrahydrone E; tonic hind limb extension

THELEP Chemotherapy of Leprosy Program (WHO)

theor theoretical

ther therapeutic; therapy; thermometer

THERAP therapeutic

ther ex therapeutic exercise

THF tetrahydrocortisone or tetrahydro F; tetrahydrofolate; tetrahydrofluorenone; tetrahydrofuran; thymic humoral factor

THFA tetrahydrofurfuryl alcohol; tetrahydrofolic acid

THM total haem mass

Thor thorax, thoracic

THPA tetrahydropteric acid

Thr threonine

THRF thyrotrophic hormone-releasing factor

Throm thrombosis

THS tetrahydro-11-deoxycortisol; Times Health Supplement

THT Teacher of Hydrotherapy

TI thalassaemia intermedia; thymus independent (cells); transverse diameter between ischia; tricuspid insufficiency (incompetence); tumour inducing

Ti titanium

TIA transient ischaemia attack

TIBC total iron-binding capacity

TIC trypsin inhibitory capacity

tid *ter in die* (L) three times daily

TIF tumour inducing factor

TIg tetanus immune globulin

tin *ter in nocte* (L) three times nightly

tinc tincture

tinct tincture

TIP translation inhibiting protein, tumour-inhibiting principle

TIRR Texas Institute of Rehabilitation and Research

TIS tetracycline-induced steatosis; trypsin insoluble segment

TIU trypsin-inhibiting unit

TIUV total intrauterine volume

TJ terajoule (SI); triceps jerk

TK transketolase; thymidine kinase

TKD tokodynamometer; thymidine kinase deficient

TKG tokodynagraph

TL terminal limen; thymic lymphoma; thymic-derived lymphocyte; thymus leukaemia; total lipids; tubal ligation

Tl thallium

T-L thymus-dependent lymphocyte

TLC tender loving care; thin-layer chromatography; total lung capacity

TLD thoracic lymph duct

TLE thin-layer electrophoresis; total lipid extract

TLI thymidine labelling index; total lymphoid irradiation

TLS testing the limits for sex (psychology)

TLV threshold limit value; total lung volume

TLX trophoblast/lymphocyte cross-reactive antigens

TM thalassaemia major; Thayer-Martin (medium); time-motion technique; tobramycin; trade mark; transport mechanism; transport medium; transport messenger; Tropical Medicine; tympanic membrane

T-M Thayer-Martin (medium)

Tm maximal tubular excretory capacity (of kidney); thulium

TMA tetramethylammonium; trimethoxyphenyl amino-propane (a hallucinogen); thyroid microsomal antibody; trimethylamine

TME Teacher of Medical Electricity; total metabolizable energy

TMF transformed mink fibroblast (cell line)

TM$_G$ maximum tubular reabsorption rate (of kidney) for glucose

TMIC Toxic Materials Information Center

TMIF tumour-cell migratory inhibition factor

TMJ temporomandibular joint

TMMG Teacher of Massage and Medical Gymnastics

Tm$_{PAH}$ maximum tubular excretory capacity (of kidney) for PAH

TMP thymidine monophosphate; transmembrane potentials; trimethoprim

TMPD tetramethyl-p-phenylinediamine

TMS thallium myocardial scintigraphy; trimethylsilane

TMV tobacco mosaic virus

TN team nursing; temperature normal; true negative

Tn normal intraocular tension

TNF tumour necrosis factor

TNG tongue

Tng training

TNM T (primary tumour), N (regional lymph node metastasis), M (remote metastasis); tumour node (lymph) metastasis

TNS transcutaneous nerve stimulation

TNT trinitrotoluene

TNTC too numerous to count

TNV tobacco necrosis virus

TO original or old tuberculin (also abbreviated OT);

target organ; telephone order; temperature, oral; tracheo-oesophageal; tuberculin ober (supernatant portion); turnover (number)

to *tinctura opii* (L) tincture of opium

TOAP thioguanine, oncovin (vincristine), cytosine arabinoside (cytarabine), and prednisone

TOC test of cure

TOE epidermatophyton; tracheal-oesophageal

TOF tetralogy of Fallot

tol tolerated

TOP transovarial passage

top topically

TOPS take off pounds sensibly

TOPV trivalent oral poliovirus vaccine

TORCH toxoplasma, other viruses, rubella, cytomegalovirus, and herpes virus

tox toxic(ity)

TP temperature and pressure; terminal phalanx; testosterone propionate; threshold potential; thymic polypeptide; thymus protein; toilet paper; total protein; transforming principle (bacteriology); *Treponema pallidum;* triphosphate; true positive; tuberculin precipitation

T+P temperature and pulse

TPA tannic acid, polyphosphomolybdic acid, amido acid (staining technique)

TPB tryptone phosphate broth

TPC thromboplastic plasma component; *Treponema pallidum* complement (fixation test)

TPCF *Treponema pallidum* complement fixation (test)

TPD thiamine propyl disulphide (prosultiamine)

TPEY tellurite polymyxin egg yolk (agar)

TPF thymus permeability factor

TPG tryptophan peptone glucose (broth)

TPI *Treponema pallidum* immobilization (test)

TPIA *Treponema pallidum* immune adherence (test)

TPN thalamic projection neurons; total parenteral nutrition; triphosphopyridine nucleotide

TPNH triphosphopyridine nucleotide, reduced form

TPO tryptophan peroxidase

TPP thiamine pyrophosphate (diphosphothiamine)

TPR temperature, pulse, respiration; total peripheral resistance

TPRI total peripheral resistance index

TPT tetraphenyl tetrazolium; total protein tuberculin

TPTX thyroid-parathyroidectomized
TR teaching and research; temperature, rectal; therapeutic radiology; tricuspid regurgitation; tuberculin R (new tuberculin); tuberculin residue; turbidity reducing
tr tincture; trace; traction; treatment; tremor
trach trachea, tracheotomy(-ostomy)
train training
trans transaction; transfer; transverse
trans D transverse diameter
transm transmission
transpl transplant(ation)
trans sect transverse section
trau trauma(tic)
TRBF total renal blood flow
TRCH tanned-red-cell haemagglutination
TRE true radiation emission
treat treatment
Trep *Treponema*
TRF thyrotrophin releasing factor
trg training
TRH thyrotrophin-releasing hormone
TRI Thyroid Research Institute; total response index (psychology); trichloroethylene
T3RIA triiodothyronine radioimmunoassay
TRIAC triiodothyroacetic acid
TRIC trachoma inclusion conjunctivitis
triCB trichlorobiphenyl
Trich *Trichomonas*
trid *triduum* (L) three days
TRIS *tris*(hydroxymethyl)aminomethane (trometamol)
TRIT triiodothyronine
TRML terminal
tRNA transfer ribonucleic acid
troch trochiscus, troche (a lozenge)
Trop Med tropical medicine
TRP total refractory period; tubular reabsorption of phosphate
Trp tryptophan
TRPA tryptophan-rich prealbumin
TrPl treatment plan
TRS total reducing sugars
TRSV tobacco ringspot virus
TRT treatment
TRU turbidity reducing unit
T3RU tri-iodothyronine resin uptake (value)

TTS   transdermal therapeutic system
TU   toxic unit; transmission unit; tuberculin unit; turbidity unit
TUB   Tubouterine (junction)
tuberc   tuberculosis
TUD   total urethral discharge
TUR   transurethral resection (of prostate)
turb   turbid(ity)
TURP   transurethral reaction of the prostate
turp   turpentine
tus   *tussis* (L) cough
TV   tetrazolium violet; tidal volume; total volume; transvestite; *Trichomonas vaginalis;* tuberculin volutin
TVC   total viable cells; triple voiding cystogram
TVD   transmissible virus dementia
TVDALV   triple vessel disease with an abnormal left ventricle
TVF   tactile vocal fremitus
TVL   tenth value layer (with reference to radiation)
TVP   tricuspid valve prolapse
TVT   tunica vaginalis testis
TVU   total volume urine (in twenty-four hours)
TW   total body water
TWA   time weighted average
TWE   tap water enema
TWSb/6   antimony sodium dimercaptosuccinate (stibocaptate)
TX   treatment; tuberculin (within cells of body)
TX   thromboxane; transplantation; treatment
TxA   thromboxane A
Ty   thyroxine; type
Tymp   tympanicity (with reference to auscultation of chest); tympany, tympanic
tymp memb   tympanic membrane
typ   typical
Tyr   tyrosine
TyRIA   thyroid radioisotope assay
Tz   tuberculin zymboplastiche
Tzn   total oestrogens after Zn-HCl treatment

U

U unerupted (dentistry); unit; unknown; upper; uracil; uranium; uridine; urology(-ologist); *utendus* (L) to be used

^{235}U radioactive uranium

U/3 upper third (with reference to long bones)

UA ultra-audible; uric acid; urinalysis; uterine aspiration

ua *usque ad* (L) up to, as far as

UAE unilateral absence of excretion

UAI uterine activity interval

UAN uric acid nitrogen

UB ultimobranchial (body)

UBA undenatured bacterial antigen

UBBC unsaturated vitamin B_{12} binding capacity

UBG ultimobranchial glands

UBI ultra-violet blood irradiation

UC ulcerative colitis; unsatisfactory condition; urinary catheter

UCD urine collection device; usual childhood diseases

UCG urinary chorionic gonadotrophin

UCHD usual childhood diseases

UCI urinary catheter in

UCL uncomfortable loudness (sound level); urea clearance (test)

UCO urinary catheter out

UCP urinary coproporphyrin; urinary C-peptide

UCPT urinary coproporphyrin test

UCR unconditioned response; usual, customary and reasonable

USC unconditioned stimulus

Ucs unconscious

UCV uncontrolled variable

UD ulnar deviation; urethral discharge; uridine diphosphate

ud *ud dictum* (L) as directed

UDC undeveloped countries; usual diseases of childhood

UDCA ursodeoxycholic acid

UDP uridine diphosphate

UDPG uridine diphosphate glucose

UDPGA uridine diphosphate glucaronic acid

UDRP uridine diribose phosphate

UE upper extremity; urinary energy

UEM universal electron microscope

UEMC unidentified endosteal marrow cell

UES upper esophageal sphincter
u/ext upper extremity
UF ultrafine; unknown factor
UFA unesterified fatty acids
UG urogenital
UGDP University Group Diabetes Program
UGF unidentified growth factor
UGI upper gastrointestinal
UGS urogenital sinus
UH upper half
UHF ultrahigh frequency
UHL universal hypertrichosis lanuginosa
U/I unidentified
UIBC unsaturated iron-binding capacity
UICC *Union International Contra le Cancrum* (International Union against Cancer)
UIMC International Union of Railway Medical Services
UIP usual interstitial pneumonia
UK United Kingdom; unknown; urokinase
UKAEA United Kingdom Atomic Energy Authority
UKCC United Kingdom Central Council
U&L upper and lower
ULN upper limits of normal
ULT ultrahigh temperature (pasteurization)
ult *ultimus* (L) ultimately, last
ult praes *ultimum praescriptus* (L) last prescribed
UM unmarried; upper motor (neurons)
umb umbilicus(-bilical)
UMMC University of Michigan Medical Center
UMNL upper motor neuron lesion
UMP uridine-5-monophosphate
UMT Units of Medical Time (Brit)
UN United Nations; urea-nitrogen
uncomp uncompensated
uncond unconditioned
uncond ref unconditioned reflex
UNCOR uncorrected
UnCS unconditioned stimulus
unct *unctus* (L) smeared
undet ori undetermined origin
Unesco United Nations Education, Scientific and Cultural Organization
ung *unguentum* (L) ointment
Unicef United Nations International Children's Emergency Fund

unilat   unilateral
Univ   university
univ   universal
unof   unofficial
UNRRA   United Nations Relief and Rehabilitation Administration
UnS   unconditioned stimulus
uns   unsatisfactory; unsymmetrical
unsat   unsaturated
unsym   unsymmetrical
UO   urinary output
UOA   United Ostomy Association
UP   under proof
U/P   concentration in urine and plasma (e.g. glucose)
up ad lib   ambulatory (patient may walk)
UPS   uterine progesterone system
UQ   ubiquinone; upper quadrant
UR   unconditioned response or reflex; unsatisfactory report; upper respiratory; urinal; urology; utilization review
Ur   urine
URA   uracil
ur anal   urine analysis
URC   upper rib cage
ureth   urethra(l)
URF   uterine relaxing factor
urg   urgent
URI   upper respiratory infection
URO   urology; uroporphyrin
uro-gen   urogenital
urol   urology(-ologist)
URQ   upper right quadrant
URT   upper respiratory tract
URTI   upper respiratory tract infection
US   ultrasound; unconditioned stimulus; United States; unknown significance
USA   United States of America; United States Army
USAF   United States Air Force
USAFH   United States Air Force Hospital
USAFRHL   United States Air Force Radiological Health Laboratory
USAH   United States Army Hospital
USAHC   United States Army Health Clinic
USAHS   United States Army Hospital Ship
USAMEDS   United States Army Medical Service

USAN   United States Adopted Names (Council)
USASI   United States of America Standards Institute (formerly ASA, now ANSI)
USB   United States Biochemical (Corporation)
USBS   United States Bureau of Standards
USBuStand   United States Bureau of Standards
USCG   United States Coast Guard
USD   United States Dispensary
USDHHS   United States Department of Health and Human Services
USHL   United Stated Hygienic Laboratory
USHMAC   United States Health Manpower Advisory Council
USMC   United States Marine Corps
USMG   United States Medical Graduate
USMH   United States Marine Hospital
USN   ultrasonic nebulizer; United States Navy
USP   United States Pharmacopeia
USPHS   United States Public Health Service
USR   unheated serum reagin (test)
USS   untrasound scanning
ust   *ustus* (L) burnt
USVB   United States Veterans Bureau
USVH   United States Veterans Hospital
USVMD   urine specimen volume measuring device
USVMS   urinary sample volume measurement system
UT   untested; untreated; urinary tract
UTBG   unbound TBG
ut dict   *ut dictum* (L) as directed
utend   *utendus* (L) to be used
utend mor sol   *utendus more solito* (L) to be used in the usual manner
UTI   urinary tract infection
UTP   uridine triphosphate
UU   urine urobilinogen
UV   ultraviolet
U$_v$ Uppsala virus
UV/P   U = concentration of solute in urine; V = quantity of urine excreted in a unit of time; P = concentration of substance in plasma (ratio = clearance of the substance)
UVA   ultraviolet light, long wave
UVB   ultraviolet light, midrange sunbeam spectrum
UVI   ultraviolet irradiation
UVL   ultraviolet light

UUN urinary urea nitrogen
UVP ultraviolet photometry
ux *uxor* (L) wife

V

V coefficient of variation; Roman numeral five (5); unipolar chest lead (in cardiography); vaccinated; valve; vanadium; variation; varnish (dentistry); vein; velocity; ventilation; ventral; verbal; vertex; very; *Vibrio* (bacteriology); violet; virgin; virulence; virus; vision; visit, visitor; visual acuity; voice; volume
v *vel* (L) or; versus; very; *vide* (L) see; vitamin; volt; *von* (Ger) of (used in names)
v- vicinal isomer
VA vacuum aspiration; Veterans Administration; visual acuity; visual aid; volt ampere
V$_a$ alveolar ventilation (l/min)
VAC vincristine, actinomycin D, and cyclophosphamide
vac vacuum
vacc vaccination
VACTERL vertebral, anal, cardiac, tracheo-oesophageal, renal, and limb (defects)
VAD Voluntary Aid Detachment
VAd Veterans Administration
vag vagina, vaginitis
VAH Veterans Administration Hospital; virilizing adrenal hyperplasia
VAHS virus-associated haemophagocytic syndrome
VAKT visual, association, kinaesthetic, tactile (with reference to reading)
Val valine
var variation; variety
VAS vesicle attachment site
vasc vascular
vas vit *vas vitreum* (L) a glass vessel
VAT ventricular activation time; visual action time; visual apperception test
VB ventrobasal complex (of thalamus)
VBL vinblastine
VBOS veronal-buffered oxalated saline
VBS veronal-buffered saline (medium); vertebral basilar artery system

VC colour vision; vasoconstrictor(-constriction); venereal case; Veterinary Corps; visual capacity; vital capacity

VCA vancomycin, colistin, and anisomycin (inhibitor); viral capsid antibody (or antigen)

VCC vasoconstrictor centre

VCG vectorcardiogram

VCI volatile corrosion inhibitor

V-cillin penicillin V

VCN vancomycin hydrochloride, colistimethate sodium, nystatin (medium); vibrio cholerae neuraminidase

VCO₂ carbon dioxide production (l/min)

VCP Veterinary Creolin-Pearson; Virus Cancer Program

VCR vincristine

VCS vasoconstrictor substance

VCU videocystourethrography; voiding cystourethrogram

VD vapour density; venereal disease; ventricular dilator; virus diarrhoea

Vd volume dead air space

vd double vibrations (cycles)

VDA visual discriminatory acuity

VDC vasodilator centre

VDEL Venereal Disease Experimental Laboratory

VDEM vasodepressor material

VDG veneral disease – gonorrhoea

VDH valvular disease of heart

VDL vasodepressor lipid

VDM vasodepressor material

VDR venous diameter ratio

VDRL Venereal Disease Research Laboratory

VDRT Venereal Disease Reference Test (of Harris)

VDS vasodilator substance; venereal disease – syphilis

VE vaginal examination; ventilation; vesicular exanthema; visual efficiency; volume ejection

VEA viral envelope antigens

VEB ventricular ectopic beats

VECP visually evoked cortical potential

VEE vagina, ectocervix, and endocervix; Venezuelan equine encephalomyelitis

vehic *vehiculum* (L) vehicle

vel velocity

veloc velocity

VEM vasoexcitor material

vent ventilator(-ation); ventral; ventricular

vent fib   ventricular fibrillation
ventric   ventricle, ventricular
VEP   visual evoked potential
VER   visual evoked response
vert   vertebra(l); vertical
VES   vessel
ves   *vesica* (L) bladder; vesicular (with reference to chest sounds)
vesic   *vesicula* (L) a blister
vesp   *vesper* (L) evening
ves ur   *vesica urinaria* (L) urinary bladder
VESV   vesicular exanthema of swine virus
VET   vestigial testis (rat)
Vet   veteran; veterinary
v et   *vide etiam* (L) see also
VetAdmin   Veterans Administration
Vet MB   Bachelor of Veterinary Medicine
Vet Med   Veterinary Medicine
VetSci   veterinary science
VF   ventricular fibrillation; visual field; vocal fremitus
V factor   verbal comprehension factor (psychology)
VFDF   very fast death factor
Vfib   ventricular fibrillation
VG   ventricular gallop; very good
VGH   very good health; Veterinary General Hospital
VH   Veterans Hospital; viral hepatitis
VI   vaginal irrigation; variable interval (reinforcement); virgo intacta; virulence; viscosity index; visual impairment; visual inspection; volume index
VIA   virus inactivating agent; virus infection-associated antigen
VIB   vocational interest blank
vib   vibration
VIBS   vocabulary, information, block design, similarities (psychology)
VIC   vasoinhibitory centre
vic   *vices* (L) times
vid   *vide* (L) see
VIF   virus-induced interferon
VIG   vaccinia immune globulin
VIM   video intensification microscopy
vin   *vinum* (L) wine
VIP   vasoactive intestinal polypeptide; vasoinhibitory peptide; very important person; Vital Initial of Pregnancy (in vitro fertilization)

VIR virology
vir *viridus* (L) green; virulent
vis vision; visiting, visitor
visc visceral; viscous, viscosity
Vit vitamin (when followed by a letter)
vit vital
VitB₁ thiamine
VitB₂ riboflavin
VitB₃ nicotinamide
VitB₆ pyridoxine
VitB₁₂ cobalamin, cyanocobalamin
VitB₁₂ᵦ hydroxycobalamin
VitC ascorbic acid
VitD₂ ergocalciferol
VitD₃ cholecalciferol (natural vitamin D)
VitE tocopherol(s)
vitel *vitellus* (L) yolk
VitG riboflavin
VitH biotin
VitK coagulation vitamin, antihaemorrhagic factor
vit ov sol *vitello ovi solutus* (L) dissolved in yolk of egg
VitPP nicotinamide; nicotinic acid
VitU cabagin or anti-ulcer vitamin
vitr *vitreum* (L) glass
viz *videlicet* (L) namely
VJ Vogel : Johnson (agar)
VKH Vogt-Koyanagi-Harada syndrome
VL ventralis lateralis (nucleus); vision, left
VLB vincaleucoblastine (vinblastine)
VLBR very low birth rate
VLDL very low-density lipoprotein
VLM visceral larval migrans
VLP virus-like particle
VM vasomotor; vestibular membrane; viomycin; viral myocarditis; voltmeter
VMA vanillylmandelic acid
VMC vasomotor centre
VMD Doctor of Veterinary Medicine
VMH ventromedial hypothalamic (neurons) (nuclei)
VMN ventromedial nucleus
VMR vasomotor rhinitis
VN virus neutralization; Visiting Nurse; Vocational Nurse; vomeronasal
VNA Visiting Nurse Association
VNE verbal nonemotional stimuli

VNO vomeronasal organ
VNS Visiting Nurse Service
VO verbal order
VO₂ oxygen consumption (l/min)
voc vocational
VOCA Voice Output Communication Aid
vocab vocabulary
VOD venous occlusive disease; vision, right eye
vol volar; *volatilis* (L) volatile; volume(tric); voluntary, volunteer; *volvendus* (L) to be rolled
vol% volume/per cent
volt volatile, volatilize
VOM volt-ohm-milliammeter
VON Victorian Order of Nurses (Canada)
VOP Viral Oncology Program
VOR vestibulo-ocular reflex
VOS vision left eye
vos *vitello ovi solutus* (L) dissolved in yolk of egg
VP vapour pressure; venous pressure; ventriculoperitoneal; vincristine and prednisone; viral protein; Voges-Proskauer (test)
VPB ventricular premature beat
VPC ventricular premature contraction; volume packed cells
VPL ventral posterolateral
VPP viral porcine pneumonia
vps vibrations per second
VR variable ratio (reinforcement); venous return; ventilation rate; vision, right eye; vital records; vocal resonance; vocational rehabilitation
vr ventral root (of a spinal nerve)
VRA Vocational Rehabilitation Administration
VRI viral respiratory infection
VRL Virus Reference Laboratory
VRP very reliable product
VS vaccination scar; verbal scale; vesicular sound (in auscultation of chest); vesicular stomatitis; Veterinary Surgeon; vital sign; volatile solids; volumetric solution; voluntary sterilization
Vs *venaesectio* (L) venesection
vs single vibration (cycles); versus; vibration seconds; *vide supra* (L) see above
VsB *venaesectio brachii* (L) bleeding in the arm
VSD ventricular septal defect; virtual safe dose
VSFP venous stop-flow pressure

vsn vision
VSS vital signs stable
VT tetrazolium violet; vacuum tuberculin; vasotonin; ventricular tachycardia
Vt tidal volume
V&T volume and tension (of pulse)
VTE vicarious trial and error (psychology)
V-test Voluter test
VTG volume thoracic gas
VTI volume thickness index
VTOL vertical take-off and landing
VU varicose ulcer; very urgent
VUR vesicoureteric reflex
VV vulva and vagina
vv veins; vice versa
v/v percent volume (of solute) in volume (of solvent)
VW vessel wall; von Willebrand factor
VWD von Willebrand's disease
VWF von Willebrand factor
Vx vertex
V-Z varicella-zoster
VZIg varicella zoster immune globulin
VZV varicella zoster virus

W

W water; watt (SI); wehnelt (unit of roentgen ray hardness); weight; west; white (response); whole (response); widow-(er); width; *wolframium* (L) tungsten; word fluency (psychology)
w watt; week; wife; with
185W radioactive tungsten
WA when awake
WAC Women's Army Corps
WAIS Wechsler's Adult Intelligence Scale
WARDS Welfare of Animals Used for Research in Drugs and Therapy
WARF warfarin
WAS Wiskott-Aldrich syndrome; World Association for Sexology
Wass Wassermann test
WB washable base; water bottle; Wechsler-Bellevue scale; weight-bearing; wet-bulb; whole blood; Wilson

Blair (agar)

Wb   weber (unit of magnetic flux) (SI)

WBA   whole body activity

WBC   whole blood cell count; white blood cells

WBCT   whole blood clotting time

WBE   whole body extract

WBR   whole body radiation

WBRT   whole blood recalcification time

WBS   whole body scan; whole body shower

WBT   wet bulb temperature

WC   ward clerk; water closet; wheel chair; white cell; whooping cough

WD   Wallerian degeneration; well differentiated; wet dressing; Whitney Damon dextrose (agar); wrist disarticulation

Wd   ward

w/d   well developed

WDHHA   watery diarrhoea, hypochlorhydria, hypokalaemia, and alkalosis

WDLL   well-differentiated lymphatic lymphoma

wds   wounds

WDWN   well developed – well nourished

WEE   Western equine encephalitis

WEF   war emergency formula

W/F   white female

WFOT   World Federation of Occupational Therapists

WG   Wegener's granulomatosis; Wright-Giesma stain

wh   whispered; white

WHAP   Woman's Health and Abortion Project

WHCOA   White House Conference on Aging

WHML   Wellcome Historical Medical Library

WHO   World Health Organization

whp   whirlpool

whr   watt hour

WHRC   World Health Research Centre

WHV   woodchuck hepatic virus

WIC   Women, Infants and Children (Supplemental Food Program, USDA)

wid   widow(er)

WISC   Wechsler Intelligence Scale for Children

wk   week

WKD   Wilson-Kimmelstiel disease

WKY   Wistar-Kyoto rats

WL   waiting list; Wallenstein Laboratory (medium); wavelength

WL test waterload test
WM Ward Manager
W/M white male
wm whole mount (microscopy)
WMA World Medical Association
WMR World Medical Relief
WMSC Women's Medical Specialists Corps
WMX whirlpool, massage, exercise
w/n well nourished
WNL within normal limits
WNPW wide, notched P wave
WO wash out; written order
W/O water in oil (with reference to emulsions)
w/o without
WOP without pain
WP wet pack; whirlpool; working point
WPB whirlpool bath
WPk Ward's mechanical tissue pack (dentistry); wet
pack
WPW Wolff-Parkinson-White (syndrome)
WR washroom; Wassermann reaction; wiping reflex;
wrist
WRAT Wide Range Achievement Test
WRC washed red cells; water-retention coefficient
WS water soluble; Williams syndrome
wt weight
W/V weight of solute in volume of solvent
WW Weight Watchers
w/w weight of solute in weight of solvent
WxB wax bite
WxP wax pattern
WZa wide zone alpha (haemolysis)

X

X cross or transverse (with reference to sections); ex-
ophoria distance; extra; Kienbock's unit (of roentgen
ray dosage); magnification sign; Roman numeral ten
(10); sign of multiplication; times (multiplication sign);
unknown quantity (symbol for); *Xenopsylla*
x axis (of a cylindrical lens)
XA xanthurenic acid

Xa   chiasma
X-A mixture   xylene-alchohol mixture (for killing insect larvae)
XAN   xanthine
Xanth   xanthomatosis
X-chrom   sex chromosome
XDH   xanthine dehydrogenase
XDP   xanthine diphosphate; xeroderma pigmentosum
XDR   transducer
Xe   xenon
XES   X-ray energy spectrometer
X-factor   haem
XKO   not knocked out
XL   xylose lysine (agar)
XLD   xylose, lysine, desoxycholate (agar)
XLP   X-linked lymphoproliferative syndrome
Xn   Christian
XO   xanthine oxidase
XR   X-ray
X-rays   roentgen rays
XRT   X-ray radiation treatment
XS   cross-section
XT   exotropia (with L or R)
Xta   chiasmata
XU   excretory urogram
XX   normal female chromosome type
XY   normal male chromosome type
Xyl   xylose

Y

Y   yellow; *Yersinia;* young; yttrium
y   year
YADH   yeast alcohol dehydrogenase
YAG   yttrium aluminium garnet
YCB   yeast carbon base
yd   yard
YE   yellow enzyme
YEH$_2$ reduced yellow enzyme
yel   yellow
Yk   York (antibodies)
YMA   yeast morphology agar

YNB yeast nitrogen base
YNHH Yale-New Haven Hospital
y/o years old
Y-organ moulting gland in crustaceans
YP yield pressure
yr year
yrs years
ys yellow spot (on retina)
yt yttrium

Z

Z atomic number (symbol for); impedence; standard score (statistic); zero; zone; *Zuckung* (Ger) contraction
Z, Z^I, Z^{II} increasing degrees of contraction
ZD zero discharge
ZDDP zinc dialkyldithiophosphate
Z-disk *Zwischenscheibe disk* (Ger) intermediate disk
ZE Zollinger-Ellison (syndrome)
ZES Zollinger-Ellison Syndrome
ZF zona fasciculata (of adrenal cortex)
ZG zona glomerulosa (of adrenal cortex)
ZIg zoster immunoglobulin
Zn zinc
Zool zoology(-ological)
ZPG Zero Population Growth
ZPO zinc peroxide
ZR zona reticularis (of adrenal cortex)
Zr zirconium
^{95}Zr radioactive zirconium
ZTN zinc tannate of naloxone
Zz *zingiber* (L) ginger

Abbreviations of Titles of the Principal Medical Journals

The following is a list of frequently cited journals, abbreviated according to *Index Medicus*. Titles consisting of only one word e.g. *Lancet*) are not abbreviated and are therefore omitted from this list.

Acta Med Scand	Acta Medica Scandinavica
Acta Paediatr Scand	Acta Paediatrica Scandinavica
AJR	American Journal of Roentgenology
Am Fam Physician	American Family Physician
Am Heart J	American Heart Journal
Am J Cardiol	American Journal of Cardiology
Am J Clin Nutr	American Journal of Nutrition
Am J Clin Pathol	American Journal of Clinical Pathology
Am J Dis Child	American Journal of Diseases of Children
Am J Epidemiol	American Journal of Epidemiology
Am J Hosp Pharm	American Journal of Hospital Pharmacy
Am J Hum Genet	American Journal of Human Genetics
Am J Med	American Journal of Medicine
Am J Med Sci	American Journal of the Medical Sciences
Am J Nurs	American Journal of Nursing
Am J Obstet Gynecol	American Journal of Obstetrics and Gynecology
Am J Ophthalmol	American Journal of Ophthalmology
Am J Pathol	American Journal of Pathology
Am J Phys Med	American Journal of Physical Medicine
Am J Physiol	American Journal of Physiology
Am J Psychiatry	American Journal of Psychiatry
Am J Public Health	American Journal of Public Health

Am J Surg	American Journal of Surgery
Am J Trop Med Hyg	American Journal of Tropical Medicine and Hygiene
Am Rev Respir Dis	American Review of Respiratory Disease
Am Surg	American Surgeon
Ann Allergy	Annals of Allergy
Ann Clin Biochem	Annals of Clinical Biochemistry
Ann Intern Med	Annals of Internal Medicine
Ann Otol Rhinol Laryngol	Annals of Otology, Rhinology and Laryngology
Ann R Coll Surg Engl	Annals of the Royal College of Surgeons of England
Ann Rheum Dis	Annals of the Rheumatic Diseases
Ann Surg	Annals of Surgery
Ann Thorac Surg	Annals of Thoracic Surgery
Arch Dermatol	Archives of Dermatology
Arch Dis Child	Archives of Disease in Childhood
Arch Environ Health	Archives of Environmental Health
Arch Gen Psychiatry	Archives of General Psychiatry
Arch Intern Med	Archives of Internal Medicine
Arch Neurol	Archives of Neurology
Arch Ophthalmol	Archives of Ophthalmology
Arch Otolaryngol	Archives of Otolaryngology
Arch Pathol Lab Med	Archives of Pathology and Laboratory Medicine
Arch Phys Med Rehabil	Archives of Physical Medicine and Rehabilitation
Arch Surg	Archives of Surgery
Arthritis Rheum	Arthritis and Rheumatism
Aust J Ophthalmol	Australian Journal of Ophthalmology
Aust NZ J Med	Australian and New Zealand Journal of Medicine
Aust NZ J Surg	Australian and New Zealand Journal of Surgery
Aust Paediatr J	Australian Paediatric Journal
Australas J Derm	Australasian Journal of Dermatology
Br Dent J	British Dental Journal
Br Heart J	British Heart Journal

Br J Ind Med	British Journal of Industrial Medicine
Br J Obstet Gynaecol	British Journal of Obstetrics and Gynaecology
Br J Ophthalmol	British Journal of Ophthalmology
Br J Radiol	British Journal of Radiology
Br J Surg	British Journal of Surgery
Br J Vener Dis	British Journal of Venereal Diseases
Br Med J	British Medical Journal
Bull Med Libr Assoc	Bulletin of the Medical Library Association
Bull WHO	Bulletin of the World Health Organization
Can J Public Health	Canadian Journal of Public Health
Can J Surg	Canadian Journal of Surgery
Can Med Assoc J	Canadian Medical Association Journal
Cardiovasc Res	Cardiovascular Research
Circ Res	Circulation Research
Clin Chim Acta	Clinica Chimica Acta
Clin Orthop	Clinical Orthopaedics and Related Research
Clin Pediatr (Phila)	Clinical Pediatrics
Clin Pharmacol Ther	Clinical Pharmacology and Therapeutics
Clin Sci	Clinical Science
Community Med	Community Medicine
Curr Probl Surg	Current Problems in Surgery
Dig Dis Sci	Digestive Diseases and Sciences
DM	Disease-a-Month
Eur Heart J	European Heart Journal
Eur J Cancer Clin Oncol	European Journal of Cancer and Clinical Oncology
Eur J Clin Invest	European Journal of Clinical Investigation
Eur J Resp Dis	European Journal of Respiratory Diseases
Eur J Rheumatol Inflam	European Journal of Rheumatology and Inflammation

Hum Pathol	Human Pathology
Int J Epidemiol	International Journal of Epidemiology
Int J Pediatr Nephrol	International Journal of Pediatric Nephrology
Invest Radiol	Investigative Radiology
JAMA	Journal of the American Medical Association
J Allergy Clin Immunol	Journal of Allergy and Clinical Immunology
J Appl Physiol	Journal of Applied Physiology
J Biol Chem	Journal of Biological Chemistry
J Bone Joint Surg (Am)	Journal of Bone and Joint Surgery (American Volume)
J Bone Joint Surg (Br)	Journal of Bone and Joint Surgery (British Volume)
J Chronic Dis	Journal of Chronic Diseases
J Clin Endocrinol Metab	Journal of Clinical Endocrinology and Metabolism
J Clin Invest	Journal of Clinical Investigation
J Clin Pathol	Journal of Clinical Pathology
J Exp Med	Journal of Experimental Medicine
J Gerontol	Journal of Gerontology
J Immunol	Journal of Immunology
J Infect Dis	Journal of Infectious Diseases
J Invest Dermatol	Journal of Investigative Dermatology
J Lab Clin Med	Journal of Laboratory and Clinical Medicine
J Laryngol Otol	Journal of Laryngology and Otology
J Med Educ	Journal of Medical Education
J Med Ethics	Journal of Medical Ethics
J Med Genet	Journal of Medical Genetics
J Nerv Ment Dis	Journal of Nervous and Mental Disease
J Neurol Neurosurg Psychiatry	Journal of Neurology, Neurosurgery and Psychiatry
J Neurosurg	Journal of Neurosurgery
J Oral Maxillofac Surg	Journal of Oral and Maxillofacial Surgery
J Pathol	Journal of Pathology
J Pediatr	Journal of Pediatrics

J Physiol (Lond)	Journal of Physiology (London)
J Psychosom Res	Journal of Psychosomatic Research
J R Coll Surg Edinb	Journal of the Royal College of Surgeons of Edinburgh
J Thorac Cardiovasc Surg	Journal of Thoracic and Cardiovascular Surgery
J Trauma	Journal of Trauma
J Urol	Journal of Urology
Med Clin North Am	Medical Clinics of North America
Med J Aust	Medical Journal of Australia
Med Lett Drugs Ther	Medical Letter on Drugs and Therapeutics
N Engl J Med	New England Journal of Medicine
Nurs Clin North Am	Nursing Clinics of North America
Nurs Res	Nursing Research
NZ Med J	New Zealand Medical Journal
Obstet Gynecol	Obstetrics and Gynecology
Pediatr Clin North Am	Pediatric Clinics of North America
Physiol Rev	Physiological Reviews
Plast Reconstr Surg	Plastic and Reconstructive Surgery
Postgrad Med	Postgraduate Medicine
Prog Cardiovasc Dis	Progress in Cardiovascular Diseases
Public Health Rep	Public Health Reports
Q J Med	Quarterly Journal of Medicine
Rheumatol Rehabil	Rheumatology and Rehabilitation
S Afr Med J	South African Medical Journal
Semin Roentgenol	Seminars in Roentgenology
Surg Gynecol Obstet	Surgery, Gynecology and Obstetrics

Some Useful Sources

Abbreviations in Medicine (Scherti). Detroit, Mich: Gale Research.

Abbrevs (A Dictionary of Abbreviations) (Stephenson). New York: Macmillan.

Acronyms, Initialisms and Abbreviations Dictionary (Crowley). Detroit, Mich: Gale Research.

Allen's Dictionary of Abbreviations and Symbols. New York: Coward McCann.

American Druggist Blue Book, The. (Contains an extensive list of Latin abbreviations and their English equivalents.)

American Standard Abbreviations for Scientific and Engineering Terms. American Society of Mechanical Engineers.

British Approved Names. London: HMSO.

British National Formulary. London: BMA/Pharmaceutical Society.

Chambers Dictionary of Science and Technology. Edinburgh: Chambers.

Chicago Manual of Style, The. Chicago University Press.

Cumulated Index Medicus. Washington, DC: US Government Printing Office. (Contains a comprehensive list of abbreviation of journals and other publications.)

Current Abbreviations (Shankle). New York: HV Wilson.

Current List of Medical Literature. Bethesda, Md: National Library of Medicine. (Contains a comprehensive list of medical abbreviations.)

Current Medical Information and Terminology. Chicago: American Medical Association.

Current Procedural Terminology. Chicago: American Medical Association.

Directory of Medical Specialists (Marquis). Chicago: Who's Who. (Contains abbreviations of boards, certificates, medical schools, national and sectional societies.)

Discursive Dictionary of Health Care, A. Washington, DC: US Government Printing Office.

Dispensatory of the United States of America, The. (Contains an extensive list of abbreviations of publications.)

Doctors' Shorthand. Philadelphia: WB Saunders.

Dorland's Illustrated Medical Dictionary. Philadelphia: WB Saunders.

Handbook of Chemistry and Physics. Cleveland, Ohio: Chemical Rubber Publishing.

International System (SI) Units, The, BS 3763. London: British Standards Institution.

Letters, Symbols, Signs and Abbreviations, BS 1991 part I General. London: British Standards Institution.

Martindale's Extra Pharmacopoeia. London: The Pharmaceutical Press.

Medical Abbreviations: A Cross Reference Dictionary. Ann Arbor, Mich: Michigan Occupational Therapy Association.

Medical Abbreviations and Acronyms (Roody et al). New York: McGraw-Hill.

Medical Abbreviations Handbook. Oradell, NJ: Medical Economics Book.

Medical Directory, The. London: Churchill Livingstone.

Medical Physics, Vol II. Chicago: Year Book Publishers.

Medical Spelling Guide (Johnson). Springfield, Ill: Charles C Thomas.

Medical Terminology Made Easy (JeHarned). Berwyn, Ill: Physicians Record Co.

Medical Word Book, The — A Spelling and Vocabulary Guide to Medical Transcription (Sloane). Philadelphia: WB Saunders.

Merck Index. Rahway, NJ: Merck.

Scientific and Technical Definitions (Zimmerman and Levine). Industrial Research Service.

Understanding Medical Terminology (Clare). St Louis, Mo: Catholic Hospital Association.

Units, Symbols and Abbreviations: A Guide for Biological and Medical Editors and Authors. London: Royal Society of Medicine.

Webster's Medical Speller. Springfield, Mass: G & C Merriam.

Webster's New International Dictionary. Springfield, Mass: G & C Merriam.

Whitaker's Almanack. London: J Whitaker.

Who's Who. London: A & C Black.

World List of Scientific Periodicals. London: Butterworths.

World Medical Periodicals. London: British Medical Association.

Symbols

℥	ounce
f ℥	fluid ounce
○	pint
℞	*recipe* (L) take
′	foot; minute; primary accent; univalent
″	inch; second; secondary accent; bivalent
′″	line (1/12 inch); trivalent
+	plus; excess; acid reaction; positive
−	minus; deficiency; alkaline reaction; negative
±	plus or minus; either positive or negative; indefinite
#	number; fracture
÷	divided by
×	multiplied by; magnification
=	equals
>	greater than; from which is derived
<	less than; derived from
√	root; square root; radical

$\sqrt[2]{}$	square root
$\sqrt[3]{}$	cube root
∞	infinity
:	ratio; 'is to'
::	equality between ratios; 'as'
*	birth
†	death
°	degree
%	per cent
γ	microgram
λ	wavelength
μ	micrometre
σ	1/1000 of a second; standard deviation
Σ	sum of
π	3.1416 — ratio of circumference of a circle to its diameter
□, ♂	male
○, ♀	female
⇌	a reversible reaction
↑ or ↗	increase, increases
↓ or ↘	decrease, decreases
→	yields or causes
→ or ←	direction of reaction

Symbols used in recording results of qualitative tests:

−	negative
±	very slight trace or reaction
+	slight trace or reaction
+ +	trace or noticeable reaction
+ + +	moderate amount of reaction
+ + + +	large amount or pronounced reaction